WWW.SQUARECIRCLEPRESS.COM

W9-BYF-667

Wobbling Home

A Spiritual Walk
with Parkinson's

Jim Atwell

SQUARE CIRCLE PRESS
VOORHEESVILLE, NEW YORK

Wobbling Home:
A Spiritual Walk with Parkinson's

Published by
Square Circle Press LLC
137 Ketcham Road
Voorheesville, NY 12186
www.squarecirclepress.com

First paperback edition 2011.
Printed and bound in the United States of America on acid-free, durable paper.

ISBN 13: 978-0-9833897-2-9
ISBN 10: 0-9833897-2-1
Library of Congress Control Number: 2011930412

Publisher's Acknowledgments
Cover design © 2011, Richard Vang, Square Circle Press.
Cover design assistance from Anne Geddes-Atwell.
Photo of Jim Atwell by Douglas Zullo.

The author's acknowledgments appear at the beginning of the book.

*To my dearest Anne,
for reasons beyond
name and number.*

Contents

Acknowledgments	x
Introduction: Wobbling Home	3
Grit Between My Teeth	6
Life Viewed from High Ground	10
Follow the River	14
A Sharp Turn in the Road	18
Chance or Plan?	21
Parkinson's Progress	25
But Was I Being Watched?	28
Where the Wild Things Are	32
Fate Takes Charge, Justice Triumphs	36
Before the Point of No Return	39
Yanked Back by the Tail	43
The Gift of Tears	47
No More Tears	51
Crimson with Embarrassment	54
Quiet Celebration	57
A Step at a Time	61
Counting by Tens	64
Put in My Place	67
No More to Build on There	70
"The Hopes and Fears ..."	73
Harrowing Times at Heathrow	77
Working Along the Border	80

Back to Baltimore   83

In Transit   85

Arm-in-Arm   91

When Cows Go Bad   95

Strangers on a Train   99

In the Winter Darkness   102

Yoked as One   106

Who's in Charge Here?   110

When a Second Shoe Drops   114

In for the Long Haul   119

High Drama by Bowen's Toe   122

"Don't look at him, Marlene!"   126

Give the Man a Medal   130

Healing Hands   134

Learning the Ages of Man   138

Dear Old Earth, Still Turning   141

Here's Your Easter Basket   144

A Vacant Place Against the Sky   148

Even in the Best of Families   150

Speaking from Deep Inside   153

All Lines Down, but Still There   157

Woof, Woof, Woof-Woof!   161

It's a Matter of Time   164

All Spill, All Feel Dumped On   167

Just Pick the Right Caterpillar   170

Fresh News From the Front   174

Heinz Kuhne, Going in Style   178

We All Live in a Hundred-Acre Wood   181

Back Among the Unaware   184

Epilogue: "Tidings of Comfort and Joy"   188

About the Author   *191*

Acknowledgments

Thanks to my dear wife Anne for bearing staunchly with me, despite her own illness; and to Dr. Paul Deringer, David White, Justin Deichman, and all my healers of body, mind, and soul. Thanks to Tom Pullyblank and Tim Wiles, and to dozens of old monastic friends; and to Doug Zullo for being such an unfailing, loving support to Anne and me. Thanks to Richard Vang of Square Circle Press; and to Mary Wright of Cooperstown, proofreader *par excellence*.

And thanks beyond words to my fellow Quakers, friends in every sense.

Wobbling Home

Introduction:

Wobbling Home

Wobbling is what I do a lot of lately. Three years after a diagnosis of Parkinsonism, and despite some fine medications, the symptoms persist and slowly grow. And so I wobble, stumble, reel, and sometimes make faces I can't control. The morning mirror can startle me: right eyebrow drooping, left eye flicking like a ship's semaphore, mouth pulled up in a piratical sneer. Sometimes that face appears in public. I only know it by the looks on others' faces.

And I fall down. So far it's been more going upstairs than down, and more onto beds and chairs than floors. I fall outside, too, though so far only onto grass and baled hay.

Before breakfast, I take Blue for his walk, first down the back lawn to open up the chicken house, then around our small west field so that he can do what a dog must do. Simon the cat, who shares Blue's dog bed by night, trots along behind us. (Cats all know that any parade's place of honor is at the end.)

Blue snuffles along the fence line, offering three-legged salutes to locust posts and weeds sticking through the fence wire. Sooner or later, by a standard I've never understood, he finds just the right spot, turns three times in a circle, and unburdens himself. "Good dog! Brave dog!" I say by way of encouragement. He appreciates this, I think; afterwards he cavorts and does a victory lap around the field.

Meanwhile, Simon has done his own morning reconnaissance, his eyes, ears, and nose attuned with an acuity I can't imagine. He's on the alert for any star-crossed mouse or vole that raises its head above ground at the wrong moment.

A few days ago, at the end of this ritual and when we'd formed up for the march back to breakfast, I fell. Don't know how or why. One moment I was walking fairly well, Blue heeling beside me, Simon parading behind. Suddenly, thud! I was down, first onto knees, then face, then onto one side.

I lay a moment, taking inventory, and found that everything still worked.

By then, Blue's professionalism had kicked in. (A registered therapy dog, he brings much joy to patients at the local hospital.) Blue rushed up and began applying what first aid he could, shoving his cold nose into my ear and lavishly washing my face.

When I got on my feet, he led me by the leash back to the house. I'd taken a jolt, muddied my pants and face, but was otherwise all right. (The sheep were in other fields, and so I hadn't dived into any left-behinds.) What to say? Falling happens.

When friends ask how I am these days, I draw on a nautical metaphor. "I'm shipping water below decks, but I'm still under sail—and pumping, pumping."

And indeed, I am still under sail, and still on course. And I hope that the second word of my title suggests how that course is charted. I'm on my trip's inbound haul. I'm steering for home.

As a Christian, I see my life itself as God's gift, and in it, everything that has occurred in its seventy-plus years. That includes Parkinson's. It's certainly nothing I'd have chosen on my own, but I know that it comes from the same loving Source as my life, and it is meant to shape the rest of it.

Still, it's not exactly the hike toward Home that I'd foreseen. Parkinson's is a clumsy traveling companion. With it holding onto me, I stutter, become confused, even get stuck in place. But never mind. On my other side I have help, strong and abiding. I'm leaning on the Everlasting Arm.

Most of this book's contents come from the weekly columns that I have written since being diagnosed with Parkinson's in 2007. They've largely been published in the *Cooperstown Crier,* a weekly newspaper in Cooperstown, New York.

To give you a sense of how I've shared Parkinson's with my newspaper readers, I've kept the columns largely as they were published, addressed to a readership that had been following me for a dozen years and more. That makes for some repetition as, writing across the weeks, I reminded readers of facts already stated; but I don't think that will distract you.

And, hoping to give you a fuller sense of me, I've mixed the Parkinsonism columns among others that reflect my life and values. Some were written pre-Parkinsonism, but most since diagnosis. Skip those if they're not needed; but since Parkinsonism is so personal and varies so from person to person, I think that you need to know who's speaking to you. This isn't an autobiography, but a lot of me is between these covers.

And last, this book is mainly for others with Parkinson's and their care-partners, but not exclusively. Much of it applies to all with a chronic disease and to all who carry the burden with them. And all of it applies to fellow pilgrims, wending their own way home. (I was a Roman Catholic Christian for the first thirty years of my life and have been a Quaker Christian for the last forty.)

And so, wobble along with me! I hope I'll be good company as you read.

Your friend Jim
Fly Creek, New York
2010

Grit Between My Teeth

You know the scene. The hero has broken free of his bonds. He's run out of the mine's mouth just as the dynamite charge explodes. The whole shaft collapses behind him. He's thrown through the air but picks himself up, unharmed. He stands, hands on hips, watching grimly as a huge cloud of dust boils out of the mine's mouth.

Last week I produced that last special effect right here in Fly Creek, right in my own backyard. Except that I wasn't outside, watching the boiling cloud. I was in the middle of it.

My adventure came while cleaning the garage. That followed, as so much has recently, from our straightening up the homestead for the approaching wedding reception. (Only weeks away!) We'd offered our property for a tent reception for a good friend.

Before tackling the garage, I'd already de-moused Anne's garden shed; her husband had stupidly left a twenty-pound bag of grass seed in there over the winter.

Mice, evidently a regiment of them, had busily converted all that seed into twenty pounds of black droppings, scattering them all through the shed. And, besides trashing the place, they'd also come to think of it as their own. This spring, Anne would step inside to find three or four mice, guards, I guess, lined up on a top shelf to chatter insults at her.

After I had shoveled out all that reprocessed grass seed, I replaced it with a liberal scattering of emerald-colored anti-mouse pellets. It was gratifying to see the fresh mouse droppings gradually turn a bilious green, then diminish in number, then vanish. As did the mice.

That job done, I turned to the garage. It houses Anne's car, my rusting truck, a red canoe, file cases, lots of tools, and two chest freezers. The last are full of vegetables, fruits, and meat, all locally raised. That makes us feel healthy, and virtuous, too.

The double garage also housed what I guess, in retrospect, was about twenty or thirty tons of greasy dirt, grit, and dust. That may be an exaggeration; but the place was truly a dump, overdue for a good cleaning by seven years or so. The floor, which of course is concrete, looked to be dirt. And every flat surface was layered with more dust than was mad, jilted Miss Havisham's wedding banquet table. (This summer, treat yourself to *Great Expectations*. She's lurking there to scare you.)

The day that I was assembling shovels and push brooms for the garage job, my neighbor and buddy Wolfgang Merk pulled into the driveway. When I said what I was reluctantly about to start, Wolf said, "Hey, there's an easier way." Wolf explained that every year he cleans his big garage/workshop in one fell swoop—with his leaf blower. He just fires up the blower, starts at the back of the garage, and blasts all the debris forward and out the doors.

What a great idea! What a labor saver! And so down to Wolf's garage we went, and back I came with his leaf blower. I gassed it up outside my garage, put on a face mask and ear plugs, headed deep into the garage. There I cranked the motor to life and pointed the muzzle down.

That's when the simulated mine explosion occurred. Wolf's idea, it turns out, is a great one for a year's worth of garage dirt. But tackling seven years' worth makes for an Oklahoma dust storm. From outside the garage, it must have looked as if the place had blown up. Inside, in the middle of it, I felt like a ladybug sucked into the vacuum-cleaner bag.

In a half-crouch, I worked grimly, blowing boiling clouds of gray dust towards the doors—or where I thought they were. For, despite the mask, I was half-blind, my eyes running and smarting. Grit stung my forehead, piled up behind my ears. Pompeii must have felt like that, just before the really heavy stuff began to fall. Half way through the job, I shut off the blower and stumbled out of the garage. Anne was out there, standing at a safe distance from the billowing cloud. "How's it going?" she asked.

Well, how to answer that?

"You should look at yourself," said Anne, smiling. I peeled off the goggles. My clothes, hands, and arms were a uniform dirty gray, like a bit player's in "The Mummy's Revenge." And when I glanced at the mask in my hand, I saw what had caused at least part of my blindness. Its lenses were dust-gray, too.

My bride, bless her, offered to take over the job at that point. But I strapped on mask, re-plugged my ears, and plunged back into the cloud. Ten minutes later the air began to clear; I could see what I was doing. And fifteen minutes later I staggered out again, the job done.

"Strip on the back porch," said Anne, always practical. I did so and padded upstairs to the shower, foolishly glancing into the bathroom mirror. Same aging body, of course, but now with gray mummy hands and arms, and with a face gray except for where the mask had fit. That part looked normal, except for the bleary red eyes. I don't know when a shower had felt so good.

I told this story to Karl Loos, the bride-to-be's father; he and his wife had come from Boston to help the couple with arrangements. Karl had his own story, a great one.

Earlier in the spring he had got out his own leaf blower, stored since the fall. Outside his garage, he yanked the cord on the blower. It roared to life and launched, over his lawn, an entire mouse nest and its residents. Squatters, they'd moved into the blower's tube for the winter. What an eviction notice!

"I felt bad laughing," said Karl, "but I couldn't help it." Hey, who could? I'm having fun just thinking of that starburst of shocked Boston mice. Those trespassers were kin to the ones who had trashed Anne's shed. As the song says, "They had it coming."

Well, I survived my own explosion. It's good to be in clean clothes and my normal color again. But, a week later, I'm still grinding grit between my teeth.

Life Viewed from High Ground

Twenty years ago, I suddenly turned into a hiker. The change was not long after my first wife Gwen's death. Maybe I was trying to out-walk the awful grief. I hiked a lot down in the Maryland countryside, along the Potomac towpath, and even some of the Appalachian Trail. I drove up to Fly Creek, New York, and hiked seasonal roads and logging trails, learning the turf of what would become my beloved new home.

On several trips abroad, I had hiked both in Wales and England, exploring the coasts and circling many of the Lake District's lakes. One day in England, high above Lake Windermere, I met an ancient ram. He stood under a gnarled tree, unmoving. The ram's head was down, with his muzzle resting on the soil. I knew the look; I had seen it in other animals.

"He's decided it's time to die," I thought. "He's come off from the flock and picked this spot. Now he's waiting."

I sat watch with him for an hour, recalling Chaucer's tale about a man who was granted a wish never to die but forgot to add that he wasn't to grow old, either. And so he aged and aged across centuries of life, and became a wizened creature bent almost to the ground. He hobbled along, tapping it with his stick, wailing, "Oh, Mother Earth, dear mother! Please let me in!"

When finally I walked away, the old ram still stood motionless, muzzle to the dirt.

Probably all my hiking, and especially my move up to Fly Creek, was my way of leaving the flock. In grief, I thought it was my time for me to be a solitary again, a monk as I had been in my late teens and twenties. I was meant to settle into the small farmhouse in Fly Creek. And wait.

But then, after seven years (bless God!), I remarried, and it turned out that my Anne loved to hike, too. With her, I've walked all around England and Wales again, and even toured the Isle of Wight. Recently, during a reprieve in Parkinsonism, I did some modest hiking in Scotland and even climbed to the top of a sheep-covered hill in Wiltshire. Oh, wondrous!

My best trek, however, will remain the one in 1990. It was 95 miles along Britain's South Downs Way, a trail along rolling hills that follow the southeast coast about five miles in from the English Channel.

One looks south and east from those heights across the coastal towns to the glinting Channel; and north and west over vistas of dark forest and of patchwork fields rich in crops of gold and green. Each distant village is marked by a church spire, its cluster of cottages and barns nestling at the crossings of narrow country roads.

My walking partner for this trip was a good friend, Michael Thrower, principal of Northbrook College in West Sussex. We were both still desk jockeys back then, and it might seem foolhardy that the two of us, middle-aged and feeling it, took on that formidable trek.

In fact, as a hike, ours was a bit soft. Mike's wife Barbara would deliver us to a starting point each morning, then pick us up in the afternoon after we'd done about fifteen miles of climbing up the flint hills and down again. Then she'd haul us home in the Land Rover to showers, supper, and bed—and the next morning deliver us to the latest end-point to start another stint.

But soft or not, by the weeks' end the hiking had us almost knackered. The last day was twelve miles, up and down more hills, to the English Channel—and then up and down the Seven Sisters, four miles of promontories that sheer off into the Channel below in cliffs of white chalk. The drop from them is dizzying, hundreds of feet onto rocks and roaring surf.

Stumbling down the last slope of the last Sister, we could see dear Barbara far below, waiting by the Rover. Inside its open boot we could also see the glint of a silver tray. On the tray, it turned out, was chilled champagne and smoked salmon on brown bread. She has a sense of style, that Barbara ...

There'd been much talk between Michael and me those seven days, but also long stretches of companionable silence. Sometimes this was for lack of breath while climbing; one of us would punch the other's shoulder to stop.

"Here, now," he'd say, "stop a moment and look back at the view opening behind us." It was a transparent strategy; we both played along with it.

But most often our silences followed on absorption in the surrounding beauty and in resulting quietness of spirit. And I know we were sharing a single thought, too. For that footpath is ancient; humans have traveled it at least since the last Ice Age.

I suspect that anyone who does that trail these days imagines a plodding file, millennia long—all the humans who've picked their way along the same track of broken chalk and flints. Iron-Age Celts traveled it, and Roman soldiers, and Picts painted blue. So did brown-robed monks and mitered abbots, armored knights and stonemasons, the Roundheads and Cavaliers, redcoats, and then Victoria's imperial troops. And, with their backs bent under their loads, centuries of farmers, herders, tradesmen, shepherds. Thousands, across thousands of years.

Twenty years ago, Michael and I trudged at the rear of that phantom column of walkers—each of whom had surely been as real to himself as I am to me. And, like me, self-important and full of plans.

In time, all in that long procession ahead of us had died,

vanished from the flurry of life as abruptly as if they'd stepped off the chalk cliff's edge at Beachy Head. Dropping away, they opened the path to Michael and me, who walked the flints and chalk behind them. And in two decades since our hiking, the line's already grown ten thousand long behind us.

All along the South Downs Way stand mossy ruins of wayside shrines, sacred rings, stone plinths, and tombs from prehistory. For people have always prayed along those windswept heights. And, I'm sure, they still do.

Follow the River

I wish you could have known him. Your life would have been enriched. And you'd probably have been in a quiet crowd some weeks ago. It filled an old clapboard church up in the Unadilla hills to celebrate his life.

During the service you might well have voiced your own memories of him. And you'd surely have joined in singing hymns he loved, especially the old gospel standard that opens, "When peace, like a river, attendeth my way." In days past, the man's superb, almost operatic baritone made that church's wooden walls vibrate as he sang the refrain, "It is well. It is well with my soul!"

Even his name was majestic: Stanford Aston Mighty. He was born near Kingston, Jamaica, sixty-seven years ago, the son of a successful farmer. He once told a group of us that as a little boy of five he was awed to discover the river that ran through the fields near his home. "I'd only known a trickle of water as it flowed from the faucet," he said, "but here was a vastness of water! It was sweeping down from somewhere, heading somewhere else."

Mesmerized by the river, the little boy set off at once to find its source. He walked barefoot for hours and for miles. Late in the day, worn out, he sat down between the river and a road running next to it. He hadn't given up his quest, but he had to rest.

Soon a farmer came along the road in a wagon and saw the little boy asleep. "Son," he said, "I know you! You're Robert Mighty's boy. But what are you doing here, so far from your home?" The answer was, of course, in the river, in finding its source. But Stanford was just too weary to explain. And so the kind farmer picked him up, set him in the wagon, and hauled him home to his relieved parents.

In telling us that story, Stanford, already dying, told us the story of his life. All his days he kept searching for the Source, never giving up on his quest. For Stanford was a mystic, a man who fervently believed that the ultimate Source can be found and embraced, immediately, in this life.

He was a committed Christian, finding the anchor of his faith in the Quaker school he attended in Kingston. With the Quakers he memorized the scriptures, and with them he learned the grand old gospel hymns.

"When peace, like a river ..." No wonder he loved that hymn best.

In his last days, Stanford told us another story, too. As a young man he earned a degree at England's Bristol University, but he also spent much time walking throughout England, especially along riversides. I've seen a photo of him from that time. In it, Stanford looks like a young Sidney Poitier: mahogany skin, piercing black eyes, high forehead and cheekbones. And like Poitier, Stanford has a look of majestic command.

Once, he said, he was hiking in the Lake District and topped a hill to face a breath-taking panorama of woodlands, fields, flocks of grazing sheep, even a distant manor house with castle ruins next to it. The magnificent scene made the young man's heart sing.

"It came to me suddenly," said Stanford. "I didn't have to own any of that! I was free of its burden, and yet it was all mine to enjoy!" And that epiphany became the touchstone of his life. He and his wife Cora, a perfect match for him, lived their life with minimal concern for possessions, maximum concern for loving service to others.

I knew Stanford through Butternuts Quarterly Meeting, the unit that links our local Friends with Quakers from Binghamton, Hamilton, the Mohawk Valley, and Unadilla.

Stanford loved sessions that brought us all together. He was a gifted cook, and when we'd finished our business meeting, Stanford and Cora would enlist the help of a half-dozen others to carry in the coolers of food they'd brought along, much of it made with a grand Jamaican flair. That big, warm-hearted man saw food as a sacrament. For him, a potluck meal was a thanksgiving, a eucharist.

If you had known him, I know that what you'd remember most today would be that astounding singing voice. It had a church organ's depth and fullness, and Stanford joyfully used it for music from show tunes to hymns to oratorios.

When, toward the end, he was bedridden and wasting slowly away, a group of us would visit to sit with him in Quaker silence, to read Bible passages, to sing. It was only at the very end that he could not raise that wonderful voice to sing with us.

Once, when I was there alone at his bedside, I was reading him some of the Psalms. Stanford was drifting in and out of morphine-induced sleep, but that didn't matter. I began to read that sad lament of the exiled Hebrews, "By the rivers of Babylon." Suddenly, eyes still closed, he sang from Handel's setting of that very psalm. In a rich, modulated voice that could have filled a theater, Stanford sang, "How can I sing the songs of the Lord on an alien soil?"

It was the song of one waiting for his painful exile to end.

And end it did, in late May, with all the beauty of spring outside his room's windows. At the funeral home in Unadilla, people wept when they saw him. In death, the years had dropped away. He looked like Poitier again, perhaps at age forty.

During the funeral, people reminisced, laughed, told their own Stanford stories. His fellow Rotarians were there, and his family doctor of many years, and wonderful relatives from Canada and downstate and, of course, from Jamaica.

At the service's close, a niece, her voice as awesome as Stanford's, burst into song. She plastered us back against the pews with a gorgeous, bluesy hymn. Then we buried him under a cloudless spring sky.

Live free of possessions, love and serve people, follow the river to its Source. He'd done the first two all his days. And finally, I'm sure, he found where that river rose. And there he surely sings, "It is well. It is well with my soul."

A Sharp Turn in the Road

I promise that I won't belabor you with this, week after week. But my Anne's reaction at the news, almost at once, was, "You have to write about this condition. Lots out there face it, either in themselves or in loved ones. You can help."

Anne's right, of course. (I always take her insights seriously, even if it sometimes takes me days to admit my agreement.) It's my plan, then, to report to you occasionally, but not so often as to change this column's tone—Scout's honor! Anyway, here's the news, plainly stated:

I've been diagnosed with Parkinson's disease.

You know, I don't much like seeing those words in type. But that's my status. I have a progressive, degenerative disease, one that's incurable. Parkinson's will share my body and shape my life for the rest of my days. But it won't become my life. Not if I can help it.

Some background: The first symptom showed up while Anne and I were in England in May, sitting aboard a southbound BritRail train. We were settling in, catching our breath, after mad dashes to make connections. We'd arrived from Liverpool in London's Paddington Station, then had to rush across the city on the Underground. We'd surfaced at vast, tumultuous Victoria Station and then had run to board a train for Chichester. We'd clambered aboard, stowed our bags, and now had a quiet ninety-minute ride south to the beautiful cathedral town and our friends' home.

Sitting there in the train carriage, congratulating ourselves for making the links, we both noticed that the fingers on my right hand were trembling. I spread them, stretched them, rested the hand on my knee, but still the tremors continued.

"Too much running for an old man," I joked, and we both laughed. But then a man sitting in front of us stood up and turned to face us. I'm guessing he was a doctor.

"Sorry to eavesdrop, friends, but I overheard what you're discussing." Then he looked steadily at me. "Don't ignore what your hand is doing. You get that checked as soon as you go home."

And of course I did, especially since the tremors re-curred several times before we were back in Fly Creek. And with them came an increase of some other oddities I'd been noticing for some months. I'd gone stumble-footed and was regularly catching my right foot on carpet edges. And my walk had become like that of a sailor new to shore-leave, one who's still shifting his weight as if he's adjusting to a rolling deck. "Sea legs," the Navy calls it.

On a first visit to my prime-care doctor, I laid out the symptoms, and he ran a series of simple in-office tests. Two weeks later I was back again and, at the doctor's suggestion, had brought Anne along. She confirmed the symptoms that she'd watched with growing concern. My doctor booked me for an MRI and sent me to a neurologist.

The neurologist gave me more tests, including a walk up and down his hallway. "Your stride is shortened," he said, "and your arms aren't swinging as you walk." More tests followed and then a later diagnosis. It is Parkinson's.

And what's that? Here's my present understanding: Mine isn't a new brain. In fact, it's long out of warranty, and replacement parts just aren't available. Well, one part of my brain's original equipment, now seventy years old, has been slacking off in making dopamine. That's a secretion that both stimulates and controls my body's movement.

A lack of necessary dopamine causes, initially, tremors, unsteadiness, and reduced motor skills. What can follow is still grimmer yet: spasms all throughout the body, speech impairment, and reduced cognitive function. As one who's lived his private and public life through communication, those last two points really haunt me.

And here's the kicker: By the time that the first visible symptoms appear, the disease may have been underway for years. At the early onset point, where I now am, dopamine production may already have slacked off by as much as eighty percent.

Just as I'm in the early stages of the developing symptoms, I'm also just beginning to come to terms with what they mean. In itself, Parkinson's isn't a fatal disease; rather, it just gradually kills a great many capacities that define us as active humans. As I said, what presently scares me most is the thought of impaired speech and, worse, a steadily dimming mind. If that gets under way, will I realize it? Maybe this column will become my canary in the mineshaft. (If it gets unreadable, please let me know.)

I've never had trouble accepting my mortality. As some grim philosopher once said, "Every life is a voyage that ends in shipwreck." Some of us settle lower and lower in the water till it finally pours over the gunwales, and down we go. Others have their hulls stove in by a metaphorical reef and dive to the bottom in no time. I've always presumed I'd fall into the second category. Traditionally, men in my family live into their seventies and then are pole-axed by a massive coronary or stroke. I'd like to continue that tradition.

And here's a lucky irony. Because I'm getting the disease so late in life, odds are that something else *will* kill me before the worst of the Parkinson's effects are upon me. (For such a mercy I humbly pray. Amen.)

OK, no more on this subject for a month or so, at least until after I've been to the Parkinson's clinic down at Johns Hopkins in Baltimore. My neurologist, God bless him, is arranging this.

Chance or Plan?

What about the swirling currents that move us through our lives? Sometimes, just like a floating leaf, we tumble over shallows and rocks; sometimes we snub briefly against a shoreline. What about those currents? Is some plan spinning itself out, or are we carried on and to the end by sheer chance?

Beats me, friends! But when I look back across my decades, I'm awed by what has brought me (so far) and has beached me happily in Fly Creek.

Maybe I'm only run aground temporarily here; maybe some errant wave will swing me out and on, down the stream. I don't think so. I believe Fly Creek, more like home than any previous place, is where I'm beached for good.

But, oh, how I got here! Here's the short form: a boy from Annapolis, Maryland, a sleepy southern town back in the fifties, goes off to become a monk. Then thirteen years praying, studying, teaching. Then two-dozen years at a fine Maryland community college as professor and dean; eighteen of them very happily married to another academic, Gwen Vosburgh.

After cancer took Gwen, a few more years at the college, and then answering an urge to move north, to what had been our planned retirement home in Fly Creek, New York. And, months before leaving Annapolis, meeting Anne Geddes, product of her own sweep of events that had carried her, south and east, all the way from Calgary, Alberta, to southern Maryland.

And then our happy marriage, already fifteen years old,

and our blessed life in our hamlet, our town, our county, our home.

It dizzies me to think back on my sweep down the stream, and the improbable surges that moved me from one setting to another. I'm tempted to change the image, think of myself as a pool ball, caroming from other balls and from cushioned sides till I come to a temporary rest—only to be rapped and sped on my way again.

Here's an example, not from my life but from Gwen's. For her childhood's events ended up defining my later life, and Anne's, too.

Gwen's dad, pastor of Edmeston, New York's Second Baptist Church when she was small, accepted a call to a church in Cameron, South Carolina. That's a village about the size of Edmeston, though its wide streets and lawns are shaded by live oaks festooned with Spanish moss, and the old houses all have deep porches and rocking chairs. The Rev. Vosburgh had moved his family a thousand miles south, from peaceful Edmeston to another village of peace.

Cameron's peace had been shattered once, though, a decade before. Sheriff George Tilley, a man in his thirties, had been called out of bed in the middle of the night. An escaped murderer had been recaptured and needed to be hauled back to the jail. A generous man and widely re-spected, Tilley dressed and headed out to do the job.

Whoever turned Willie Gideon over to Sheriff Tilley had not properly searched him. Out on the highway, though in handcuffs, Gideon pulled a pistol from his boot and shot Tilley. The mortally wounded sheriff was found in his wrecked car. Rushed to the hospital, he died soon after. Gideon was later caught, still in his handcuffs, and returned to prison, now to face a second murder charge.

That story was already legend in Cameron when the Vosburghs and their three daughters arrived in town. And the sheriff's widow, Miss Johnny Tilley, as everyone called her, rocked on her front porch as the Vosburgh girls played around in the shaded yard with her own adopted niece Nancy.

The Rev. Vosburgh, by all accounts, was a selfless pastor; he took on two poor country churches as well as his Cameron charge. And he was a witty man and a practical joker, too. But strong of will, he began to lock horns with his oldest daughter as she entered her teens. That was my Gwen.

When Gwen was fifteen and the tension was high, the pastor still carried on a practical joke that had long since become old hat. He'd come in, exhausted from his schedule, stagger towards the bed, and fall on it, gasping and holding his chest. "This is it! Goodbye all! I'm gone!"

This act had long since brought only a dismissive "Oh, dad!" from the girls and his toddler son. But one dark evening he fell on the bed, gasped, and fell silent. It was ten minutes before they realized that this was no joke. He was dead of a coronary.

My Gwen, shocked, grieved, and guilt-ridden that she'd somehow caused this, ran screaming into the moonlit streets. People poured out of houses; and down her own porch steps came Miss Johnny, the dead sheriff's .38 revolver in her hand. If something awful was happening again, by God, she was going to stop it!

Gwen ended up moving north again to spare expense to her widowed mother, two sisters, and a baby brother—and perhaps to flee undeserved guilt. She lived with Edmeston's Chesebrough family, who generously financed her first years in college. Gwen eventually earned an MBA, taught first at Alfred, and then was recruited down to Anne Arundel in Maryland, the very same year a young ex-monk joined the faculty.

That's how an awful night in Gwen's childhood changed the current of her life, made it overlap with mine, and brought me to Otsego County. From grief over her death, I later fled north, too.

Mere chance or plan beyond grasping? I don't know. But, sharing life with dear Anne, who gave me life again, I'm awed, humbled, grateful.

Parkinson's Progress

Time, I think, to report on how Parkinson's disease and I are doing in our joint venture. I'll hold to my promise of not belaboring you with this topic; but an occasional report, I hope, will be a kind of public service. I'm not the only one who finds himself rowing this boat.

In fact, after I told you about my diagnosis, I had a half-dozen phone calls from men around here, all of them with Parkinson's. Some have been dealing with it for years, and all were wonderfully supportive. But a couple of them, it seemed, have withdrawn from life and into their homes. They don't want to be seen with what once was called "the shaking palsy."

That's too bad, though I readily sympathize. Every time Anne and I eat out, I dread splashing soup onto the table-cloth, or coffee into my own face as I raise a cup. Once Parkinson's has joined the family, it's like taking an unruly child to the restaurant. You can stay on the alert, but there's no predicting the results.

But, back to my report. No need to bury you in facts and figures; if you're wired into cyberspace, megabytes of material are available literally at your fingertips. Just couple your search engine to "Parkinson's," and it will haul a train-load of information onto your screen. But here's a quick summary.

Parkinson's is progressive, degenerative, and, at present, incurable. Its primary cause is a brain's reduced dopamine production, which functions like a governor in controlling bodily movement. Whence the quakes, shakes, and spasms that are its most obvious symptoms. Parkinson's also affects speech, swallowing, posture, walk, balance, and even facial expressions. The current treatment addresses the symptoms. Research, advancing rapidly, is aiming for the cause.

Over a half-million Americans have Parkinson's, and doctors turn up an added fifty thousand of us each year. Though it's not much comfort, the rich and famous are among us. Perhaps the best-known Parkinsonian is Michael J. Fox. After being hit with the disease at age 30 and at the height of his film career, he has turned his energies to education on the subject and to fund-raising for research. And in Muhammad Ali you see some classic symptoms of advanced Parkinson's: his muted, slurred speech; his robotic movement; his face, once so antic, turned into a rigid mask.

But all that information, as I say, is readily available to you. What I can provide is a sense of how the disease feels to someone you already know well through these columns. I can tell you about Parkinson's from the inside. And when I raise the subject here every few months, it will be to do just that.

In a recent column I said Parkinson's was a creature now sharing my body and life. I'm past personifying the disease that way, as if it were some alien that had invaded me. I guess it speaks to our primitive past that we brand diseases as assaults from the outside. We say, "I've been hit by a rotten cold." Or, "Poor guy suffered a stroke," as if it were a literal blow. Or, "She suffered a heart attack at sixty-five." Or, "He was stricken by pneumonia."

From terrible personal experience, I understand the tendency to see disease as an attacker, an invader. As my first wife's body and life were consumed, I came to hate her cancer as a willful creature. I thought I could sense its powerful malevolence, and I cursed the cancer for what it was making Gwen suffer through. When, at the end, she died in my arms, that hatred even cut through the searing grief. I heard myself growl, "You've killed her, you bastard, but at least now you'll die, too!"

But, personifications aside, many diseases do enter us from the outside. They come, not as willful demons, but as bacteria and viruses, mindlessly indifferent to us, mindlessly in search of a host organism. Or perhaps they arrive as environmental toxins, insensible to the havoc they will wreak on healthy organs.

But Parkinson's isn't like that; and acceptance of the fact is my biggest challenge these days, the one that I want to share with you. Though some research suggests that toxins can get it started or speed its progress, Parkinson's is essentially a brain breakdown. It's the failure of my original, factory-installed equipment, with really nobody and nothing outside me to blame.

Parkinson's starts deep in the basal ganglia, the part that's called "the primitive brain" because we share it with all sentient creatures. Deep down in there, the steady secretion of dopamine slows drastically as production cells die off. That's bad news, since, as I've said, dopamine is the governor that checks and controls bodily movement.

Yep, that's what spatters the soup on the tablecloth or splashes coffee into one's own face. That's what causes the stumbling walk.

The effect of this knowledge on me is strong. I'd really sooner have someone, something outside of me to blame. But there's no blame to be assigned, even to me. It's just that a major function of a very complicated organism is breaking down, and I'm deeply involved. The organism is me.

Here's my present image for myself: I'm driving at night through blowing snow and sleet. I'm miles from anywhere. But I'm behind the wheel of a good, steady car that I know well; and I'm drawing a lot of comfort from that fact. Then, without warning, the motor begins to miss and sputter, the whole car to buck. That, friends, is about where I am.

But Was I Being Watched?

Recently I was inveighing to you against too-smart machines elbowing into our lives to advise or even order us what to do. I'll offer one more offensive example. Then I'll tell you of the worst interaction I've had with such machines, at least to date.

I used to teach with a colleague who hated machines that acted human. He was especially outraged by ones that flashed "Thank you" after you'd done what they demanded. Automatic toll-takers were his special target. Whenever he pulled up to a toll plaza that flashed a demand for seventy-five cents, he'd throw the money into the metal funnel, but always in nickels and dimes. Then, before the machine could count it, he'd burn rubber and barrel through the red light before it could shift to "Thank you."

"Take that!" he'd shout with great satisfaction as the machine triggered its alarm bells and then choked them off. "Have a nice day!" he'd add, glowering in the rear-view mirror.

Don't know where that guy is now. Jail, maybe.

These days, of course, we have E-ZPass, which, pointless misspelling aside, does get us through the gates a lot faster. But I think the affront to us humans is even greater: The state-sponsored electronics now talk, not to me, but right past me and directly to my car. I have no idea what my windshield unit says to the tollgate unit; I'm not party to their conversation. But when they're done, the gate flashes, "THANK YOU." I guess those words are directed to me since it's switched to human language. Grinding teeth, I drive away, feeling like a chauffeur for that thing stuck to my windshield.

I know, that's over-reaction. But now let me tell you about my capstone humiliation by smart machines, at least to date.

A few winters ago, Anne and I were driving down to Baltimore-Washington Airport to catch a flight to England. We were behind schedule and in a Poconos snowstorm. We both wanted to grab some lunch, and both of us needed a bathroom.

"Look, how's this for a plan?" I asked, squinting my way through the blowing snow. "We can't waste any time. So I'll pull into the quick-stop at this next exit. You run in, order the sandwiches, then head for the bathroom—there's only one. I'll pump the gas, and come in for the john as you're paying up."

Phase one of the plan worked fine. But men of my age will understand what happened out at the pump. As soon as the cold wind hit me, there was a sudden surge in my urge. And when I pressed the nozzle trigger and the gas began to gush, there was no more deferring. I had to go. ASAP.

In an instant I'd surveyed the scene. I was forty feet from the store and on the far side of our car. No traffic was passing. Snow was blowing in a near white-out. Could I get away with it? I tried to buy time with a kind of two-step from foot to foot. No use. No choice.

I switched the gushing nozzle to my left hand, and, after some frantic fumbling with the right, got through my clothes. And then—yes, friends. The present writer stood there in the snowstorm, emptying one tank as he filled the other. As much as possible, he faced away from the store and discolored the snow against one of the posts of the gas pump's canopy. Many a passing dog had done the same thing, he rationalized; and, besides, the blowing snow would soon cover the evidence. But what, he wondered, would the next sniffing dog think?

In the middle of things, a wind gust snatched his cap from his head. He'd have tried to grab it, but he was out of hands. Luckily, the cap wedged against a trash can. Oh, my.

When I'd gotten both jobs done and all equipment stowed, I felt pretty hang-dog myself. My cap retrieved and head down, I plowed through the snow and into the store, heading, not for the john, but to the counter to pay for sandwiches and gas. The short woman behind the counter grinned as I walked up. Her smiley-face badge said, "Hi! I'm MADGE."

"Lord, that snow's fallin' like a house afire! Could you see what you was doin' out there?"

"Barely," I said weakly.

Anne walked up just as I turned from the register and started for the door. She looked a bit puzzled. "I thought you had to …"

"I'll explain," I said, and held the door for her. I hope that the door, closing behind us, muffled Anne's shouted "You did WHAT?" and her peals of laughter. I didn't glance at that canopy post as I got in and drove us away.

We made the plane, were safe aboard and airborne when I leaned back and began rehearsing that scene. Suddenly a chill came over me. What if I were wrong? What if something had been watching my antics?

Security cameras! Just about every gas station has them to catch gas thieves. Oh, Lord! What if some machine's beady eye recorded every phase of my pitiful clown show? That meant the counter lady could have watched it all on her monitor. I drew in a sharp breath. Had hers been a knowing grin? Was that why she had asked, "Could you see what you was doin' out there?"

I sank deeper in the airplane seat and imagined slow days in the store, customers coming in, some local calling out, "Hey, Madge, show Billy the old fool pumping gas and peeing in the snow! It's a hoot!"

Heaven help me if there's ever an "America's Funniest Security Tapes." Madge will send it in, for sure.

Where the Wild Things Are

When we drove around the Otsego hills in my pickup, my old buddy Arrie Hecox most often sat in silence, his face set in his all-purpose scowl. But he was having a good time. In his mid-eighties, Arrie loved to ride along, just looking. He saw each vista not just as it was just then, but as he'd known it across four score years.

Driving along in silence was just fine with me; I've a taste for quiet. There was always something to think about, most often the next week's column. But sometimes Arrie would yank me out of my reverie. Inside that closed cab, he'd nearly stop my heart with a sudden shout.

"COWS!" he might bellow, if he'd spotted some interesting ones. Or, more often, "STOP!" That might mean a pause for him to climb out and answer nature's call. More often, it meant that he was seeing something special on what looked to me like a thickly wooded slope.

"House stood right there," he'd say, pointing. "A barn was over there, milk house, corn crib, sheds. Good orchard, too." Short pause, then gruffly, "All that work! All gone!" The last was my signal, after my own respectful pause, to let out the clutch.

A farmstead gone, indeed. Nothing left, in among the trees, except perhaps a cellar hole and a few rotting fence posts. All that brutally hard work—dropping trees, dragging out stumps, shifting rock by the ton—all undone by re-claiming nature. For if we humans ease off our clearing, nature doesn't waste time. In twenty years she's closed things over again.

That's why our Otsego County is now far more wooded than it was a hundred years ago. And with the woods' return, something else is coming back, too. Some native wild things, driven north into the Adirondacks as their habitats were bared, are back again. So far, they're in small numbers. But to us country folk, their return brings unease. Some of those creatures feed on smaller animals, including livestock and pets.

A friend up Fly Creek Valley was shocked to pull in her drive and see a bobcat sitting right on her front porch, licking its paw and grooming like a big kitty. A really, really big kitty; bobcats can run to sixty pounds. Gray, it was, with spots of black. At the car's approach, the cat was gone in four graceful bounds.

Hunters this year also claimed to see a few even bigger cats—the kind that Natty Bumppo called "painters," and we call panthers or cougars. These cats can weigh one hundred fifty pounds, and they can leap fifteen feet, up and into a tree. Luckily, they try to stay away from humans. But they like livestock, and also dogs and cats.

I think about such animals each time I let Owen outside. Owen is fourteen, but he could still scamper up a tree ahead of a pursuing fox. But a pursuing bobcat would be right up the trunk after him.

And then there are bears. Black bears. A lot have been sighted this past year, and last month one of them raised holy hell with Paul Lord's beehives. Please, put Pooh Bear out of your mind. This wasn't a small, dear, slow-witted blunderer. This was a full-grown male, a loner, shambling along at over three hundred fifty pounds. And the brains that Pooh pretended to have? This bear really had them, in spades.

Paul and his wife live high up in Pierstown. A big retired Marine, Paul loves the delicate, patient work of a beekeeper, loves working in tandem with the bees, turning part of their work into splendid raw honey. In good years, sales of it are important extra income.

This could have been a good year, but that big bear wiped out any chance of it. Its destruction eclipsed all profits and reduced productive hives by forty percent. In total, it ate perhaps four hundred pounds of pollen and honey.

The bear's rampage started almost under the Lords' bedroom window. It tackled a shed full of rectangular comb frames and reduced them to sticky kindling. After a second attack there, and a third, Paul installed a motion detector that emitted a high-pitched shriek. That drove the bear off, but it shifted the search-and-destroy operation to the next hilltop, where a dozen of Paul's beehive boxes are clustered in a field.

In summer that field is like an airline hub, with thousands of bees winging through the sunshine from every direction, each heading for its own hive as if for a hanger, each waddling inside to unload leg pouches of nectar. To the huge hungry bear the site wasn't an air hub; it was a commissary. It shrugged off shock and bee stings to crash through the charged fence and knock over the hives.

When, after the first assault, Paul upped the fence's current, the bear took to reaching between the wires, swatting a hive with his paw, and knocking all or part of it through the fence.

Night followed destructive night, and the bear refined his technique, standing up, reaching over the fence, and delicately lifting the top off the hive box, exposing the vertical line-up of comb frames. It figured out fast that the cold made the bees cluster in the center frames. And so the bear, using claws as large as a man's thumb, would carefully lift out an outer frame, carry it away, and sit down to lick it clean of contents. Then it would return for another.

After a month of such damage, the bear was finally brought down, but not by Paul Lord. A neighbor about a mile away was walking some woods with his rifle when he spotted the giant on his hind legs, supplementing his honey diet with shriveled apples still on an old tree. The hunter dropped him, and destruction at Paul's place ended.

I think I just heard some tender soul say, "Poor bear! He was only trying to feed himself!" Well, yes. As was Paul.

"But bears were here first!" I'm not sure what to make of this argument except to repeat that bears and some other wild things, having gone north for a while, seem now to be back. I don't think that means we have to leave. It does mean, however, that there will be confrontations.

If we share this turf, we'll have to live with one another. But if I see a bobcat anywhere near my lambs ...

I'm a Quaker, but I pack heat.

Fate Takes Charge,
Justice Triumphs

You usually get a present from me about this time—something to wind up the year and celebrate the fun I have in talking with you each week. Choosing is not always easy. It's job enough to find a suitable gift for even one friend or relative—you just try getting one for a whole readership.

But I've succeeded. I went back over the past year's notes, looking for stuff I hadn't already shared with you, and found an entry of two words: "umbrella justice." That recalled a vastly satisfying incident. I hope it'll bring you as much delight as it did me.

It happened on a hot day last summer in a pleasant restaurant on Cooperstown's Main Street. More precisely, it occurred behind the restaurant, in the shady fenced garden that is the place's warm-weather annex. Around noon, Anne and I were seated toward the back of the garden, sharing the ambiance with quiet diners at a half-dozen other umbrella tables.

One table toward the front was empty for a while. But then a party of three entered from the restaurant. The two adults were dressed in yuppie-tourist mufti, right down to pricey leather waist pack and camera case. In their late thirties, they had a quiet, self-assured look. With them was a small barbarian of about four.

I say "barbarian" because no one, it seemed, had made a step toward helping that little boy become civilized. As his parents, smiling indulgently, settled themselves at the empty table, their ruffian ran amok among the other ones, glaring up into people's faces and staring into their plates. After a few moments of this, his mother said sweetly, "Austin, wouldn't it be nice to come sit in your chair?"

After her third repetition, Austin made a final face at a diner and frog-hopped toward his parents. He clambered onto his chair seat and then stood on it, legs spread, hands on hips, as if daring a challenge.

"Wouldn't it be nice," his father said evenly, "to sit in your chair while we tell you about the menu?"

In answer Austin snatched up a menu, opened it, and clapped it on his head like a roof. Then he pivoted to check reaction from other tables. When no one smiled or laughed, he slapped the closed menu down on the table, and then hoisted a bent knee onto it.

"I wonder if the table is a good place to put your ..." His mother got that far before Austin, grabbing the umbrella shaft for support, swung the second knee onto the table. Smiling a bit grimly, the parents grabbed the table's edge to steady it.

"Now, Austin," said the dad, "maybe it's time to settle down and talk about lunch." But Austin, still kneeling and clutching the umbrella pole, had found something far more interesting. It was the umbrella latch, about halfway up the pole.

The restaurant's umbrellas, it turns out, are ingenious. They're designed, not to fold down around their poles, but to slide, fully open, straight down to protect the table from a sudden shower. This was demonstrated when Austin, with a yank, released his umbrella's lock.

Oh, what a good moment! First came a muffled "Thwoop!" The sound drew every eye toward that front table—where Mr. and Ms. Permissive and rowdy Austin had suddenly disappeared. That colorful umbrella had dropped like a candle snuffer—extinguishing the whole unpleasant scene. Some few around us gasped. Most laughed in delight.

Two waitresses scurried to the table and raised the umbrella back up the pole. From under it, frozen in tableau, the family re-appeared: parents bent forward over the place mats, Austin still on the table, but on hands and knees. All were open-mouthed. As a waitress apologized to his tight-faced parents, a pale boy eased off the table, into his seat. And for the rest of the meal, while his parents ate in silence, Austin's decorum was perfect.

So there's my year-end gift to you—assurance that, sometimes, at least, fate steps in and straightens out human behavior. And does it with good humor.

At the end of a mean-spirited year, when good order has routinely been roughed up in high places, I find that comforting. Hope you do, too.

Before the Point of No Return

Back in Annapolis twenty-five years ago, I lived in an all-electric sub-division. Even then, the monthly bills were getting astronomical. My neighbor Bart once grieved to me about the cost. He shook his head slowly and said, "The only way more extravagant to heat your house than by electricity is to set fire to it."

Tragically, Bart's ironic line now has global application. Burning the house you're living in: That is the very kind of absurdity, writ terrifyingly large, that marks our steadily destroying the planet as we live on it.

But, more precisely, we're not destroying the planet. It is, after all, a ball of inert rock. What we're destroying is the delicate film of living matter that veils its surface. That film is composed of living species, inert matter raised to fragile, temporary life as fish, trees, dragonflies, eagles. The delicate film encompasses all creatures, great and small. Among them is our human species, the one that supposedly knows what's going on. But despite our vaunted braininess, we are the only species that seems hell-bent to undercut all living things. We're the ones sawing the limb upon which we're all sitting.

But that's not the rocky globe's problem. It has suffered surface crises worse than the one that we're causing. Barring really big asteroids, the planet itself will likely last eons till the sun gutters, then blows up. And so, even if we manage to wipe out ourselves (and, with us, countless thousands of blameless, beautiful species), just give the globe twenty millennia or so to undo the damage we've done to its water, soil, and air. Then it will carry on just fine. Without us.

A glum prophet in the 19th century said, "Mankind is a disease the earth has caught. But don't worry. Earth will get over it." How sad if we prove him right. How sad if we cure the earth by our self-destruction.

But how did we get into such a mess? Well, some of western civilization's oldest stories offer a symbolic explanation. I mean the creation stories, right at the beginning of Genesis.

No telling, of course, how old those stories really are. The oldest part of Genesis was shaped by countless generations as oral tradition before being first written down around 2,900 years ago. But whatever the stories' age, or whether you see them as factual history or inspired parables, those stories nail down fundamental truths about us and our link to the earth.

For instance, one story shows the Creator molding a first human from the earth's soil, shaping the mud before breathing life into it. That story says that our oldest ancestor, short of God, is the planet itself. It says that we don't simply walk the earth's surface. We're made from it. We're an integral part of nature itself. We are of it, in it, sustained by it. (A Native American tradition echoes that story movingly. "Mankind," it says, "is earth that has sat up.")

The Genesis stories also point up our link to the earth in another way—in God's first directive to his new humans. Gesturing to the paradise in which they've been placed, the Creator gives a command: Tend this place.

Well, I guess that hasn't worked out. (Was God the first, I wonder, to shake His head and say, "Where do I go to get good help"?) In fact, we haven't been tending the place. We've been trashing it, right from the get-go. For, make no mistake, past generations showed no more respect for the earth than we do. This present, perhaps final, crisis follows on two facts. First, there are now so frighteningly many of us: Half the humans who've ever lived are alive right now. And second, in recent centuries we've grown very skilled at plundering and at exploiting the planet, even as we largely ignore the consequences.

In fact, we deliberately blind ourselves to those consequences, denying them angrily even as the evidence mounts. Why? Because to acknowledge the consequences would mean facing the need to rein in sharply the "American Dream" that mass communications have now made humanity's dream: unlimited personal goods, comfort, and convenience, all snatched at greedily through manic consumerism. We're addicted, you see, and don't want to think about withdrawal. But as a prophet might say, woe upon us if we don't wise up.

Sorry about the sermon, brothers and sisters, but the point can't be made too strongly. Just now, there are many nightmares afoot to haunt us—our mindless, misguided wars, for instance, plus the explosive growth of wild-eyed, worldwide terrorism that they have ignited.

But beyond those horrors, there's the most awful nightmare of all, the one that should have us sitting up, sweating and wide-eyed in the night. It's the wreck we're making of the planet. That fact should keep us awake—and something else, as well: We're seeing the first, undeniable signs that earth, speaking through a battered Mother Nature, is beginning to defend itself. It's beginning to strike back. To cast off the afflicting disease. Us.

As important as is the seeking of peace, triumph over wars and other outrages will be moot if all the players get swept off the board.

Again, sorry for my harangue. But take note, please, that my intent isn't specifically religious. It's based in rock-bottom practicality. We can't continue messing in our own nests. Sawing off the limb we sit on. Burning down our house to heat it.

We need (and now I'm borrowing an old religious term) to convert. That literally means to "turn away from." From what, we know in our hearts; but towards what? We know that, too. But do we have the will?

Yanked Back by the Tail

Look out, here comes an update on my Parkinsonism. It won't be unduly gloomy, but I have to talk about human frailty. And so, if spring's final arrival would have you sooner thinking of daffodils, forsythia, and robins bobbing on your lawn—well, you might want to skip over to the sports pages.

Centuries ago, monks working on manuscripts often had a steady companion on their desktops, staring back at them from empty eye sockets. It was a long-empty human skull, often that of a monk from centuries before. This ornamental companion was called a *memento mori*, a reminder of mortality. In case the point be missed, sometimes the skull carried a brief inscription: "As you are now, so once was I; as I am now, so you will be."

In other words: "Monk, use your brief years well; ages hence, all that may be left of you is your own yellowed skull on someone else's desk, with his spare quills stuck casually in your eye socket."

I don't want this column turning into a *memento mori*. But I've been talking with you as friends, each week for so many years, that I think you want to know about the changed life evolving in me. That's presumption, I know; and if I'm wrong, make haste over to the sports pages. There you'll find the excellent reporting of Eric Ahlqvist, who's been conversing with you even longer than I have.

It's two months since I talked to you about coming to terms with Parkinson's, and much has happened in that time. I've learned, for instance, that this notably subjective disease has an erratic pattern in me. Some days it's in charge, some days I am. That's why you may see me striding along Cooperstown's streets as effortlessly as I used to, and other days see me depending heavily on a cane.

My first steps each morning tell me who's to be in charge that day.

The big event of those two months was the visit down to Johns Hopkins. Anne and I took Blue along on the trip as a cheerful distraction, leaving him with dog-lover friends when we drove into Baltimore and the University Hospital.

Hopkins is huge, sprawling over many city blocks. The outpatient clinic fills a whole block itself, a charmless six-story concrete monolith. Two cops were directing traffic out front as cars and vans dropped off patients. Lots of oldsters; lots of crutches, walkers, canes. Anne dropped me off there and headed for the equally massive garage across the street. (She was five times up and down the corkscrew ramps, top to bottom, before she found a parking place.) I joined the group funneling toward the entry.

The entry was a revolving door eighteen feet wide. In deference to the clients, its panels swept around slowly, shepherding in one group as, on the other side, they dismissed another back onto the sidewalk. I shuffled in with six others, half watching for a sign saying, "Charon's ferry, straight ahead."

No such sign inside, but a vaulted marble lobby, echoing with voices and cell-phone rings. As I stood uncertainly, patients passing me to left and right, a warm voice spoke from behind a counter.

"First time here? Let me help you." Behind the counter was a middle-aged man in suit and tie. His skin was a rich ebony, his smile serene and comforting. "You just tell me where you need to go, and we'll hand you on, right there."

Suddenly at ease, I told him I wanted the Neurology Center. "Piece of cake!" he said, laughing. "Four floors up. Just step down this counter to that nice lady. She'll take some information and head you to the escalators." I did and then sat down across the lobby to wait for Anne.

From my seat I watched the man who first greeted me. He studied each group swept in by the revolving door, watching for anyone who stopped and looked around uncertainly, as I had. I saw him call over several and send them along, reassured. Talk about the right man in the right job!

As the appointment time neared, Anne was still circling around and around, up and down, over in the garage building. And so I boarded the elevator alone. The car looked dingy and worn, as did the fourth floor carpeting, reminders that this was a big-city hospital. No way to keep it as clean and gleaming as our Bassett Healthcare always is.

At the Parkinson's Clinic, more helpful people. And here came Anne, a little harried from her garage adventure. We sat for perhaps ten minutes, and then a tall, white-coated man greeted us by name. It was Dr. Zoltan Mari, an internationally-known specialist. He'd come out to meet us and lead us to his office. His smile and handshake were warm, but as he walked up to us, his intense eyes were appraising me. The consultancy had already begun.

We spent an hour and a half with Dr. Mari, who retested my reflexes, my balance, my coordination. He questioned both Anne and me closely and listened attentively to our answers. At the end he stated his agreement with everything done for me at Bassett, adding, "The medicine you are taking is what I would have prescribed, had you first come here."

This kind man walked us all the way back to the waiting room and, shaking hands warmly again, said, "I will send my report to your doctor. He and you must feel free to phone me here, anytime." We headed down to the lobby, feeling we had a wonderful new ally on our team.

Back at Bassett, we agreed with the neurologist that I'd stay on the same medication as long as the Parkinson's did

not overwhelm my ordinary life. And so my present pro-
gression, with me some days in charge, PD calling the shots
on others. And for a blessed ten days recently, the symptoms withdrew completely, only to return afterwards.

What's this feel like? Well, sometimes it seems I'm a
mouse in the grip of a playful cat. It tosses me around and
repeatedly lets me run away, thinking I've escaped. Then it
shoots out a paw and yanks me back by the tail.

The Gift of Tears

A couple of weeks ago in the quiet of Quaker meeting, two thoughts rose in my mind and drifted like smoke in and through each other. They're related, but I'm not sure just how, except that both are bittersweet and speak of human frailty. With your presumed permission, I'm going to try to sort them out here. I'll tell you the first event this week. You'll have to hang around a week for the second.

The first thought was memory of an event that occurred seventy years ago in a building now burnt down, among people long dead, and in a subculture almost gone itself. The building was Ammendale Institute. It was the novitiate, or boot camp, for young men entering the Christian Brothers. I did my own basic training there in the mid-1950's, but the event I'm going to recount lived as legend among monks who were novices in the late-1930's—about when I was born.

Back then, as in my time, Ammendale housed three distinct groups. The first was a small high-school prep, consisting only of boys who thought they wanted to join the order. Then there were the novices, eighteen and nineteen years old, who after three months at Ammendale as postulants, were given their habits and religious names and began the official year and a day of novitiate. The novices typically numbered about thirty, half in a group just starting their year, the others just finishing up.

The third Ammendale population was composed of retired brothers, mostly in their seventies and eighties, worn out from decades in the classrooms of elementary and high schools, a boys' reformatory and an orphanage, and a college, all run by the Christian Brothers. Most of the old monks were ambulatory and attended services downstairs in the chapel. Others, either wheelchair-bound or too frail to handle flights of stairs, joined in community prayers and meditation from the choir loft across the back of the chapel.

Some of the elderly monks were still very keen-minded, and these entertained the novices with great stories of dealing with crowds of unruly students, not to mention truculent pastors and tyrannical bishops. Others of the retired moved in the mists of early dementia. Their actions provided a different kind of diversion for the young novices.

Among the downstairs monks was a Brother Azarias. He was well into his eighties back in the 1930s, and dead long before I entered Ammendale. But his name lived on among the novices of my own time because of a strange thing that overcame him in his declining years.

Azarias had read deeply into the lives of the saints, accounts of men and women who had lived lives of heroic sanctity in ages past. He was most fascinated by very colorful figures of the third to sixth centuries.

There was, for instance, St. Simon Stylites, who spent decades doing penance on the top of a twenty-foot pillar, often standing on one foot. (The little food that he ate was hoisted to him in a bucket; he sent down wastes in the same container.) Other penitents rolled in thorns or encouraged ants and scorpions to bite them. Some endured blistering heat, and others freezing cold, all in penance for the world's sins and their own.

Viewed across a thousand years and more, we might think of such penitents as *bona fide* wackos; but not so Brother Azarias. To him they were models of virtue to be admired and emulated. He was especially taken with saints who had been given "The Gift of Tears." These were men and women so overwhelmed by a sense of sinfulness that they wept copiously and almost constantly. Some developed channels down their cheeks created by the salty flow.

So impressed was old Brother Azarias that the Gift of Tears seemed to descend on him. He felt so unworthy of it that he wept bitterly—though only a couple of times a week and only during morning meditation in the chapel. This was a major distraction to the novices, but a useful one; they kept themselves awake in anticipation of it.

Each time the Gift struck Azarias, its progress was as predictable as Old Faithful. First the chapel silence, normally broken only by the occasional clank of the steam radiators, carried a long and wistful sigh. Then, just about a minute later, a long, choked moan filled the air. (By now the novices were biting their lips, digging fingernails into palms to keep from giggling.)

Next Azarias produced a prolonged wail, starting at mid-scale and sliding chromatically up an octave or so. Then came the geyser of tears: loud blubbering, open-mouthed and top volume. (At this point an occasional novice would slide to the floor, gasping with laughter. He usually didn't last much longer as an apprentice monk.)

But no one, of course, challenged Brother Azarias. Though some thought he was deluding himself, indulging in performance art, the majority stance was that the seeming Gift of Tears might just be the real thing. And it's not smart to fool around with Gifts from God.

A smoldering exception to the majority sat above Azarias' head in the choir loft. Brother Jeffrey, a wispy little man wheelchair-bound and almost lost in his black habit, had known his confrere Azarias for over sixty years. He had actually been a novice with him, back when that same chapel was lit by gas fixtures, and the building's long corridors by coal-oil lamps.

Truth be told, Jeffrey had never liked Azarias; he'd always thought he was shallow and melodramatic. And a morning came when the bravura performance below the loft became too much for Jeffrey. He wheeled his chair forward, right against the rail. He leaned over and boomed down in a voice like God's from Mount Sinai:

AZARIAS, YOU OLD FOOL!
SHUT THE HELL UP!

And with a gasp and gulp, Brother Azarias did. His Gift of Tears disappeared, and for good. Afterwards, meditation became a time of silence, but far more of an ordeal for the novices, who had to struggle to keep their heads from nodding and their knees from slipping off the kneelers. And for Brother Azarias, it became a time of bitter sadness, though he couldn't cry over it. He had no tears anymore, of any kind.

Those two old men died within a couple of months of each other, Azarias first, then Jeffrey. After the earth was tamped down on Brother Jeffrey, I can almost imagine him shifting in his casket, turning a cold shoulder towards his confrere of sixty years. But then, perhaps rancor ends with death. I'd like to think so.

No More Tears

I was telling you friends the bittersweet story of old Brother Azarias, a monk in the order to which I belonged for thirteen years. Azarias was long dead when I did my novitiate as a Christian Brother, but stories of his bizarre behavior still hung in the novitiate's air, a quarter century after his death.

For Brother Azarias was given, or had convinced himself that he had, the Gift of Tears, a blessing from God far more common early in Christianity's first millennium than near the end of its second one. The Gift held that some chosen souls, so stricken at the thought of the world's sinfulness and their own, would weep incessantly, even constantly, to the point that furrows developed down their cheeks to carry off the salty flow.

Azarias, as I said, became convinced that he had been granted the Gift of Tears; and two or three times a week he disrupted the silence of morning chapel meditation with his sobs, gasps, and juicy blubbering. He was finally silenced when another old monk shouted out for him to shut the hell up. And that was the end of Azarias' Gift of Tears. He died a few years later.

I dug that story out of my memory banks because it's a fascinating glimpse into a separate world, a world now so changed as to be almost unrecognizable. And also because the story is tangled into my present Parkinsonism.

I promised you I'd tell you about Parkinson's progress every few months to give you something of a unique perspective on it. For I'm writing, not as someone outside, researching the disease, but inside, living it.

Back in April I last talked to you about sharing mind and physical being with Mr. Parkinson. (I guess I could have said "Ms. Parkinson" instead, but that might have suggested unseemly thoughts for an aging, happily married man.) Parkinson and I continue to share every moment of every day, and part of every night, too.

The last-mentioned is a change since April. I'm now awakened most nights, often more than once, by my hands flapping at my sides as if I were trying to take flight from the bed. Sometimes it's only my fingers that are in wild motion, mimicking someone typing at about 150 words a minute. An episode lasts about three or four minutes, and then stops. I'm beginning to think that the cause is in the previous day's medication finally wearing off.

By and large, that medication is pretty effective in controlling Parkinson's behavior in me. I can raise a cup or glass to my lips with fair success, but I usually end up bringing the left hand into play to steady the right. And I can type on the laptop so long as I keep close attention to what I'm doing. For my days of multi-tasking are over. I must be single-minded. Always.

Parkinson's, as I've said, gradually erodes the accumulated habits of a lifetime—the ones that allow us to do thousands of activities without thinking of them. In fact, we carry through much of our life on automatic pilot, successfully doing complicated things without any real attention to them. Thus we drive cars, change diapers, climb stairs, wash dishes, pop sugar peas from their pods.

All those useful habits are housed deep down in our primitive brain, sometimes called our "reptile brain" because we share the basic survival capacities with creatures down to and including the scaly and the cold-blooded.

But when Mr. Parkinson does his job on the neurotransmitters that are based down there, what were automatic processes must be shifted up to the brain's frontal lobes and become conscious and deliberate. And I'll tell you, friends, that's a tiring business. Coupled with constant tremors, it's exhausting.

And here's the kicker: though my daily medication holds at bay the most debilitating symptoms, when I get very tired, the symptoms come storming over the defenses. I'm dropped like a stunned horse.

So life becomes a campaign to eat right and exercise so as to build up energy and stamina, and then to husband those values and apply them to what I really want to do, or to what really must be done.

You'd think the frustrations of such a pattern of life would have me often in tears, but it never does. For that's something else that's changed since my column last April. Whether it's the disease or the medication, something fundamental has changed in me.

I can't cry. About anything. Ever.

I can't judge Brother Azarias' Gift of Tears, but I've lost the gift of the ordinary, everyday kind. And it makes me feel an odd kinship with an old man dead before I was born.

I first realized the change in me when Anne and I carried a lifeless Owen (Simon's predecessor) out of the veterinarian's office two years ago. Losing that cat, my close companion for so many years, should have torn me up, had me sobbing. I *was* torn up. But no tears came. And none have ever since.

The urge, the need to cry will rise, fill my chest, swell in my throat. But then, like thunderheads that promised rain but drop none, the emotions move on, leaving me unrelieved, choked.

I don't want to be overdramatic, but treasure your tears. Ordinary tears that follow on pain or loss or grief, are a precious gift. Somehow they purge pain that could otherwise be unbearable. That gift is no longer mine. And I can't even cry about it.

Crimson with Embarrassment

A Saturday back in 2006 found our Fly Creek pastor a conflicted man. The Reverend Thomas Pullyblank had promised his son that they'd go to Oneonta to see "Flushed Away," and the little boy was bouncing with excitement about it. But that very afternoon, said Tom, he'd be missing Michigan versus Ohio State, the football game of the decade. Maybe he'd see "Flushed Away," but he'd miss the Clash of the Titans.

I share lots of values with Parson Tom, but not his football passion. Down in Annapolis in my boyhood, we guys gave a lot of time to fishing and hunting and swimming and sailing, but not as much to organized sports. Further, I was a nerd, a bookish sort. And so I grew up a football illiterate. I understood the game and of course was taken by the town's mass hysteria when Navy played Army, but I never had Tom Pullyblank's passion for the sport.

And passion it is. Growing up in western New York, Tom watched football from his crib and, I take it, was hurling his teddy bear down imagined fields while in diapers. In school he played the sport with real success; now, with some years on him, he still has an ex-player's zeal for the game.

By Tom's testimony, Michigan and Ohio State are presently the two best teams on cleats, and their rivalry is old, fierce. Some say it dates back to an 1803 land war that ended with Ohio wresting a narrow strip of turf to itself and taking possession of Toledo, Michigan. No shots were fired during the struggle, but both sides had militias marching up and down the narrow strip, pushing and shoving, blustering and threatening.

This ancient fray, it appeared, was to be reenacted last Saturday afternoon on the parson's TV screen, right in his living room. But he, for love of his son, would be in Oneonta, watching cartoon figures and hearing, among others, Kate Winslet do manic voice-overs. Poor Tom was torn.

Well, mine is a tender heart; I couldn't stand the man's pain. And so I agreed to tape the game for him. In retrospect, I should have offered to take that great little kid to "Flushed Away." My taping skill ranks right down there with my tackling and quarterbacking. Still, Saturday afternoon found me in my living room, on the couch. The game's TV audience was later estimated at 21.77 million. I'm in that figure someplace.

As you'd imagine, I'd been very careful as I inserted the tape, tuned the set to CBS. At least two other stations were carrying big games, too. One of them was the Iron Bowl, Auburn versus Alabama in another ancient grudge match. I had paused on that channel to watch the camera pan across the masses of screaming southerners and thought affectionately of Bill Yancey. He was a fellow dean back at my college, a fussy old bachelor whose life's passion was the Alabama team. If someone joked about them, Bill would sputter and his neck and face would bulge and turn scarlet. We called it, of course, "the Crimson Tide."

Good old Bill had an autographed photo of Bear Bryant on his wall; if he hadn't been Baptist, I believe there would have been votive candles in front of it. Well, he's long gone now—died in a nursing home of a stroke. I wonder if he was watching a game.

Anyway, I got everything set, turned on the recorder, and settled onto the couch, the sound turned down, a book in my lap. The wood stove was radiating warmth. Anne was at the other end of the couch, also reading. Owen the cat was curled up between us. I'd glance over randomly at the players in red and white, running and smashing together.

It happened sometime in the second quarter; I'm not sure how. When Anne and I want to avoid blaming one another for some mishap, we usually put the finger on Owen or Blue the dog. This time I think it really was Owen's fault. He stood, stretched luxuriantly, and lay down again. On the remote. And that Owen switched the channel from Michigan/Ohio to Auburn/Alabama. With the sound turned down, I never noticed. Those good ole boys were also uniformed, respectively, in red and white.

But things got worse. As the wrong two teams came up on their half time, the recorder whirred and stopped. I heaved up, leaped off the couch and to the set. The tape had run out, but no worry. I had another blank at hand, ready to insert. But the machine wouldn't let me. Following its own programmed will, it rewound—and then began to inch forward again, dutifully deleting all the advertisements. No button I could push, including "OFF," could divert it.

At just that point the phone rang. Anne took the call, sitting on the couch. And so I couldn't say any of the appropriate words. I had to sweat bullets silently through the whole damned halftime show while that machine mindlessly plodded along with its task. Then, just in time, it finished and released controls back to me. I shot in the blank tape and fell back in relief on the couch. And the recorder ground on, recording the wrong game, the wrong guys in red and white.

When he returned the tapes, Tom broke the news to me kindly, though I think his eyes were brimming. That was my turn to be swept by a crimson tide. He's a generous man, Tom, and will forgive me. I'm not sure I will.

Quiet Celebration

I was over in Clinton, New York, recently and drove past the Kirkland Art Center, which faces out on the village's beautiful green. Sight of it brought back memories of a meeting there about twelve years ago. Quakers from this part of New York had gathered there to celebrate the 300th anniversary of Quakers in the state. They celebrated in typical fashion, very quietly.

I'm not sure how many Quakers are in New York now, though no where near as many as in, say, the 19th century. Then, Friends' meeting houses dotted the countryside. Local meetings were often stops on the Underground Railroad, and their buildings offered platforms to the era's leading abolitionists and, later, to the major figures in the women's suffrage movement.

These days, some groups still gather in old meetinghouses, but others use public buildings or private homes. Our Cooperstown Friends usually meet, through the kindness of the Presbyterians, in their parish house on Church Street; though on the first Sunday of each month we join with other regional groups in meeting in the fine little clapboard church down in Emmons, kindness of the United Methodists there.

I remember very well that Clinton meeting from twelve years ago. Friends from as far away as Binghamton converged on the local Arts Center, bearing covered dishes and wicker baskets for a communal meal after worship. Then, after visiting a bit as does any gathering congregation, they settled into some folding chairs arranged in a circle on the polished wooden floor. And in moments, a calm, profound silence settled over the whole group, even over the children in attendance.

I should note that a large segment of Quakerism, especially in the Midwest, holds church meetings similar to those of evangelical Protestantism, though always with a place for silent prayer. On the upper East Coast, however, the majority of meetings are wholly silent.

My own pilgrimage has had me worshiping as a Quaker for forty years, but I'm still awed by the quality of this quiet. It's not that people have retreated deep inside themselves, leaving an empty silence outside them. Rather, the silence is something that wells up from them and flows outward to embrace the group. It is a silence of shared attentiveness, expectancy. At its most intense, in what Quakers call a truly "gathered" meeting, the quiet seems almost separate from the group that produced it—far more than the sum of its parts. It's a presence that gathers in and melds the group.

This silence follows on the most basic tenet of Quakerism, perhaps the only one all these highly individualistic spiritual pilgrims share. There is, they say, "that of God" in every human. And hence, for them, the first place to seek the divine is not in ritual or sermons or hymns. The kingdom of God, they say (quoting a very reputable source), is within you, and the place to seek God is there, within, beyond any human words or gestures of worship.

This tenet is not a denial of others' ways of worship, much less a condemnation. It is simply the Friends' way, their witness.

Scholars of religion have a name for spiritual questers who seek direct contact with the divine—without the mediation of organized religion, clergy, or ceremony. They call them mystics, and scholars say that they appear in every major religious tradition. In essence, Quakers are undramatic, matter-of-fact mystics, but of an unusual kind. For, besides their silent worship, Friends are best known by their work for peace and for the poor, the imprisoned, and those savaged by war.

Most Friends that I've met shape their spiritual questing inside the general Christian beliefs of a creating Father, a loving Christ who can raise us out of our selfishness and provide a path back home, and an abiding Spirit, one that enlightens that very path. Other Quakers, I am sure, would not even use the word "God" to denote what they're reaching for. They might say, if asked, that the reality they seek can't be captured in any finite word.

"God," one once wrote with depth and simplicity, "is that toward which I journey."

So the journeying, the worship, is done wordlessly. But not entirely. For the silent Quakers, who have no clergy, minister to one another during worship. They believe that the spirit that gathers the worshipers into silence may also speak to them through one another. And so in the course of an hour's meeting, two or three might speak quietly, voicing the fruits of their own thoughts or prayers. Such speaking is almost always brief, simple, rich in meaning. And when each voice is done, the embracing silence closes again behind it, as does still water when a hand is withdrawn from it.

And that's the way the Friends gathered in Clinton celebrated their three hundred years. As I sat there in their midst, my own thoughts ranged to other public celebrations I've attended.

I've been on the Mall in Washington, for instance, on a hot July Fourth night, among tens of thousands of happy, jostling, slightly-crazed celebrants, their excitement heightened dizzily by bands, orchestras, choruses, artillery salvos, and, finally, the anticipated mammoth, dazzling, deafening fireworks display.

I've been in stone-vaulted cathedrals at Easter, at liturgies that were a feast for all the senses: banks of lilies and blazing candles, cloth-of-gold vestments, swirling, sweet-smelling clouds of incense, processions of robed choristers, stained glass brilliant with sunlight, solemn chant, glorious polyphony, and thundering organ music with deepest pedal notes that were more than just heard, but vibrated up the length of one's spine.

I wondered at the contrast as I sat with the celebrating Quakers, drawn into the profound calm of the silence. It was good to be there.

At the end of the Clinton worship meeting, the Friends had risen and joined hands briefly, then moved to another room and tables laden with simple, delicious food. That leisurely meal seemed to me as close as Friends come to ritual. The food, prepared in their homes, was passed and shared among them, along with conversation and much laughter.

And surely more than food was shared. As much as in the worship service, a bond among Friends was being celebrated. It felt to me like a Quaker communion service.

They seem to know a lot about communion.

A Step at a Time

Time to tell you again about Parkinson's and me. I haven't mentioned the former since August. A good deal has happened, including an anniversary. Anne and I noted it, if we didn't exactly celebrate it. It's now been over a year since I was diagnosed with the progressive, degenerative, presently incurable disease. So what's been going on?

I won't bore you with a detailed description of Parkinson's; you can pull that up on the web if you're interested. My contribution is to tell you, who certainly know me well after all these years, how the progress feels from the inside. And so, here's the skinny:

I've lost more ground. I'm depending much more on a cane and I am really, really careful on steps. I'm prone to fall down. Sometimes I have trouble swallowing food. Much of each day I lose to sleep. And still I'm tired, tired all the time.

And, because my aging gray matter has largely cut production of the neurotransmitters that allow us to move through so much of our lives on automatic pilot, I must be absolutely single-minded as I do something as elemental as walking or cooking or brushing my teeth. If I'm distracted, I'll get diverted. And that can be dangerous. Oh, and I forgot to tell you that I forget things, lots of things, some of them important.

Those last paragraphs sound whiny, neurotic. So let me counter them at once by adding that I'm at peace and in good spirits. And in the most important ways, I'm still the old me, though working a lot harder at staying that way.

Let me tell you about two rear-guard actions that have

helped me greatly—and to encourage other "Parkies" who may have delayed using them to do so, and at once. For, in the case of both, the sooner is literally the better. Urgently so.

The first is physical therapy. My neurologist and friend Paul Deringer said early on that PT could help a lot with my gait and my stumbling. The former had reduced itself from a three-foot stride to shuffling along a foot at a time. The latter problem, stumbling, followed on not raising my right foot properly and put me in danger of serious falls.

By great luck I was referred to Michael Quinn, who heads Bassett's fine PT staff in their center on Railroad Avenue. A smiling, soft-spoken man, Mike immediately inspires confidence that he can help; and he does, with great effect. Through exercises in the center and others he prescribed for the Sports Center pool, Mike brought back my stride and reduced both my stumbling and imbalance. Bless him for it!

Dr. Deringer also arranged appointments with the Bassett speech therapist, explaining that my voice's loss of volume has the same cause as the shortening of my gait. Parkinson's, it turns out, plays hob with all sorts of calibrations set way back in our early childhood, including ones that control speech volume and the simple act of walking.

David White, the speech therapist, is as skilled in his field as is Mike Quinn in physical therapy; and he has the same gift for inspiring immediate confidence. David's office is on the third floor of the patient-care building. His greeting there was always warm and full of enthusiasm for what can be done.

David's first move was to show me how soft my voice had become, which he did with a sound-volume meter he placed on the table between us. He told me to match his volume as he spoke. In short order I saw that whether I was speaking conversationally, increasing my volume to lecture-room level, or shouting as if outdoors, in each case I was ten decibels below David's volume—the volume I thought I was matching.

With David's training, I've re-calibrated my sense of my own sound volume, though when I carry on conversation now, I feel as if I'm shouting. Never mind; to others, it sounds normal. Who would have thought?

Enough for now. In sum, I'm still the same Jim who's enjoyed talking to you each week for a dozen years or so. I'm that guy, but with some challenges.

I'd like to pretend I don't need help, but sometimes I do. And so, if you see me having trouble with a curb or positioning a chair to sit in it, don't hesitate to offer help. I won't be offended, rather very grateful. And I'm not a bit hesitant to accept a supporting arm on an icy sidewalk.

Counting by Tens

Sometime back, I turned seventy, made it to the classic "three score and ten." Well, you know how my head works by now; the event sent me skimming back over the years like a barn swallow after mosquitoes. Except that I had more regularity in my flight. I swooped down and landed briefly at the start of each decade. I'd picked up that habit sixty years ago in Sister Maretta's fifth grade classroom.

I'd spent the year before with Sister Alowine, a nun surely yanked out of the order's retirement home and into active duty to meet a sudden one-nun shortage at St. Mary's, Annapolis. Looking back, I'm guessing that she was about eighty; rheumy eyes peered at us from the shadow of her order's elaborate headpiece.

But she didn't miss a thing unless she slipped into a doze. That sometimes happened on sunny afternoons when she had us working on drawing maps or solving long divisions. We'd hear a faint snort and look up to see her, head dropped forward, lips fluttering. The miracle was that we behaved at such times, kept right on with our work. Maybe we had some real sympathy for the old girl—but maybe it was because she could snap awake very suddenly.

Only one of us dared make fun of her, and not of her naps but her loose upper plate. I've told you before about the plate, and the odd mid-sentence grimaces Alowine would make to reset it when it slipped. Sometimes grimaces wouldn't do, and she'd labor to her feet and face the blackboard to do serious readjustments.

When she did that, wicked Jack Pantalino, who was

always made to sit in the front row, would swing out of his desk to face us in a crouch, thumbs pressed up against his molars. He'd push up on them, miming terrific effort that made his eyes cross and seemed to lift him off his feet. At the first sign on our faces that Alowine was about to turn around, Johnny would put a hand on his desk and swing himself back behind it.

He was good at such things, was Johnny. I'm guessing he's probably in Sing Sing now, or maybe locked up on Devil's Island.

Forty years after all this, I heard the distinction young Brits make among their very elderly. In the first class are "the Wrinklies," nursing their ailments and talking too much about them. These morph into a group that totters along at grave's edge. The British kids call them "Crumblies."

Alowine was most definitely a Crumbly. I think if someone had slammed a door loudly behind her, she'd have dissolved into her original dust, leaving only a rumpled pile of black serge and starched white panels. But she was an old dear, and she did well by us. God rest her, I say.

The next year, when I was ten, I sat before a very different kind of nun. Sister Maretta was probably in her mid-thirties then. I'm guessing that she came from a big Irish family, for she genuinely liked us kids; though she held herself with a nunly aloofness. She was tall and slim, and when stood before us, arms tucked in sleeves, she was the model of sereneness. But then when she stood on tiptoe to write at the top of the blackboard, or when she swooped gracefully to pick up a piece of broken chalk, she brought a surprising new pleasure to me.

Once on the playground, wicked Jack said idly, "Wonder what Maretta looks like without her clothes?" I was horrified, but couldn't free myself of the thought. But when, agonized, I told the old priest in confession, I heard him suppress a laugh. "That's all right, son, just don't encourage the thought. Now, have you done anything really bad?"

I was crushed. My biggest sin to date, and he'd dismissed it as not even calling for absolution!

But, finally, to my point. Sister Maretta, standing hands in sleeves one day, was talking about our lives ahead. "This year all of you will turn ten. But think another ten years ahead. You'll be out of high school, some working, some in college, some of you married with children." That last one brought laughter, but Maretta went on.

"Ten more years and you'll be thirty—that will be 1968. And in 1978, forty; and 1988, fifty and probably with grandchildren." More laughter, but Maretta's narration was almost getting us dizzy. "Then 1998, then 2008 and you're seventy years old!"

Well, I'm there, Maretta, and looking all the way back to your classroom. Thank you for the practice of measuring in decades. It lets me now see the forward sweep of my life: monk, teacher, ex-monk (I decided that in 1968), college professor and administrator, eighteen years happily married to Gwen, seven years a widower, eleven years happily wed to Anne.

And I'm really sorry about those unworthy thoughts of you naked. But had you known what was going on behind that little boy's brown eyes, I'm guessing you'd have reacted like that kind old priest in the confessional. You'd have given a hearty Irish laugh.

God bless you and rest you, Maretta. I owe you and your sisters more than I can say.

Someone did say, and with considerable authority, that the greatest love is to give up one's life for others.

All of you did.

Put in My Place

I try to report to you every time I make a fool of myself. I mean it as a service, since it lets you think, "Well, at least I'm not that dumb," or, more kindly, "Jeez, I know how that feels!" Anyway, here are two fresh examples.

I swim three times a week at the Sports Center, paddling laps and doing exercises. I put on a pair of the Center's swim fins, which make me feel like Donald Duck as I flap to the pool's edge. But once in the water, I turn into Aqua Man from the comic books of my youth. He was one of a set of specialized super-heroes that have since disappeared.

There was Elastic Man, who could stretch his arm down and around the corner of a city block to nab and drag back a bad guy. And The Torch, who, when needed, burst into flames and blazed across the city skies. On contact with evil, his specialty was incineration.

But it's Aqua Man that I become when I Donald-Duck my way down the steps and into the water. I launch into my laps at superhuman speed, or at least far faster than an overweight Atwell should be able to go. It's exhilarating, and bad guys had better stay out of my lane.

Well, a few weeks ago I was zooming up toward the pool's north end when my Aqua Man radar spotted trouble. I dropped duck feet to the bottom and stared at the big room's northwest corner—squinted, really, since my glasses were back in the locker room. In the corner, half behind a big cabinet and a pile of Styrofoam floats was a slumped human figure in swimming trunks. It was motionless.

"Probably a lifeguard, taking a break and a short

snooze," I thought as I Aqua-Manned my way south again. This time I was on my back so I could enjoy my gratifying wake. Aqua man rules! But when I turned north, I began to worry.

"You know, people die from heart attacks that way—they slump down, and people think they're dozing. And they die!" I dropped my duck feet again and squinted hard at the corner. The man hadn't moved. Time to call out to the lifeguard. "Hey," I shouted, "is the guy in the corner all right?"

The lifeguard, an affable sort, glanced toward the corner and said, "That dummy? He's OK." And he went back to reading, maybe a superhero comic book.

Swooshing south again, I felt reassured. That must be a lifeguard on break, and the on-duty guy must know him since he jokingly called him "dummy." But after my turn and half back down the pool, I slowed and dropped duck feet again. "Hey, wait a minute," I thought. The superhero rescue mode was fading fast.

I paddled right up against the edge of the pool and squinted really, really hard. Hard enough to see the slumped guy's arms were articulated at shoulder, elbow, wrist, knee and ankle.

Yikes! "That dummy" *was* a dummy, the rescue dummy they use in training water safety.

Maybe it's the monastery still alive in me, but at times like that I feel compelled to confess my stupidity to some-one. And so, flapping out of the water, I duck-footed up to the lifeguards—two of them, since the one I shouted at was going off duty. I laughingly told them of my mistake. They dismissed it as an understandable mistake. Kindly, they didn't laugh till I had taken off my Donald Ducks and flat-footed it into the locker room.

The second incident involves those turkeys we're rais-ing. The three of them, big birds now, generally behave themselves as free-rangers, limiting themselves to the acre of fenced field outside their house and, with some encouragement, going inside to roost at night.

All three of those birds still think I'm their mother, but something worse is at work with one of them. If I put a chair near their shed and sit down to watch them, she'll jump onto my lap, sit down, and coo at me. That's creepy enough, but the other day she spotted a dark spot on my forearm. Sure it was a bug, she gave a lightning peck, removing the spot and a perimeter of skin as neatly as a dermatologist.

When I come into the back yard now, she flies over the fence and follows me around. And one day last week I woke from an afternoon nap to hear her whistling and cooing under my window.

I am being stalked by a turkey, you see, and there's no restraining order against such a thing. (There I go again, confessing something humiliating!)

I get no help from Anne, of course. She just laughs.

No More to Build on There

Here's a farm adventure, friends, from a few years ago when we were still having our ewes bred in September and welcoming newborn lambs in early spring. My dread always was that the ewes would start birthing at night in a snowstorm or in a power failure. My adventure didn't occur in either, but the lambs did start aborning while Anne was on a trip. I was alone.

On St. Patrick's Day morning I checked on the three ewes, then drove to the Fly Creek General Store for coffee and human company. In the time I was away, Rachel had birthed three handsome black lambs. And that afternoon, Sophie showed why she had been so enormous. She produced her own set of triplets, two black and one white.

Six lambs in five hours gave me a harried day—setting up separate pens in the shed, drying off the newborns, hanging heat lamps, trimming umbilical cords, supplying the new mothers with warm water. This was my first time facing all that without Anne's help since our marriage, but I got the jobs done. And despite a lot of rushing about, I still got to enjoy the mother's interaction with the newborns.

They sing to them. As soon as the lambs' faces clear of mucus, they begin to bleat. The mothers answer them with a soft, chuckling sound from the back of their throats. That's a special sound, heard from them at no other time. What then develops is a lilting call-and-response between the newborns and their wooly dams. It's beautiful, and I was fool enough to cry every time it happened.

The lambs are up on their long, unsteady legs within

minutes of birth, fumbling around their mothers' sides, instinctively looking for their first meal. They keep on bleating until they blunder into what they've searched for. Then they're quiet as they drink, tails wagging in pleasure. But the mother continues that soft chuckle, sometimes leaning around to lick a newborn's back.

The third of our ewes was young Tess, a last year's lamb. She had yet to deliver; and of course this would be her first time. She's been frightened and confused by all the sudden furor in the sheep shed; and maybe confused, too, by what's going on inside her. So Tess is skittish and given to sudden lunges toward the door and safety outside. But she's a flock creature, and after a time, she forces herself to come back in.

Two days after the births, I took down the bonding pens. The two new mothers now could rove the shed, with lambs crowding each one like tugs pushing against an ocean liner's sides. Poor Tess doesn't know what to make of these small, antic creatures. It's clear that she doesn't find them cute.

Nature, sadly, doesn't much care that lambs are cute, either. She's benignly indifferent to their fates. The solitary white lamb I found dead on St. Patrick's evening; it had been lain on by its mother. And the next morning I found one of the second set of triplets lying stiff and lifeless, no cause obvious. Two brief lives ended, after barely knowing light, warmth, smells, sounds, and sweet drink.

Death is a fact of life for farmers, even amateurs like me. Over the years I've been tending animals, I've faced it repeatedly, and often with the sheep. So far, the worst time involved bottle-feeding a newborn lamb rejected by its mother. The feeding went on for days, every four hours. But despite the efforts, the feeble little ram steadily weakened and slipped into real distress. And so, after trying for days to continue that life, at the end I had to stop it. That was very bad, very hard.

I guess there was a lesson of some sort in seeing each of the St. Patrick's Day mothers tending her two survivors, already indifferent to the small corpse in the same pen. It set me reciting Robert Frost's "Out, Out ..." in my mind. (That title echoes Macbeth on life's frailty: "Out, out, brief candle! Life's but a walking shadow ...")

The Frost poem used to shock my students, not so much because of its tragic subject, but because of its laconic last pair of lines. The plot is a simple one. A young farm boy is out in the backyard, cutting stove wood with a buzz saw. His sister calls him to supper, and, in his instant of distraction, the saw takes his hand.

They carry the boy in and lay him on the kitchen table. The country doctor "put him in the dark of ether." But "the watcher at his pulse took fright. No one believed. They listened at his heart. Little—less—nothing!—and that ended it."

Then come the final lines, the ones that first shock, then move one to nod sadly. "No more to build on there. And they, since they/ Were not the one dead, turned to their affairs."

That's the lesson of those two new mothers, turning their full attention to the still-surviving lambs. The mothers were alive and had duties to the living. And so they turned to their affairs.

But it's harder for humans, isn't it?

"The Hopes and Fears ..."

What an odd, lackluster buildup to Christmas it's been this year. That is, what a lackluster buildup to America's Commercial Christmas, the kind that's almost smothered the event we're supposed to be commemorating.

The event was an unusual birth twenty-one centuries ago, one that took place in abjectly poor circumstances but, according to accounts, also involved a chorus of angels and reverent visiting kings. Much of the western world came to agree that it was an event worth celebrating. But somehow, especially in these times and this country, Mammon got the upper hand and turned the commemoration into an all-star tribute to him.

You remember Mammon? The word's really just a common noun in Aramaic; it means "wealth and treasures," but of a kind and amount to choke one's spirit. The term was a handy one, and soon mammon became personified: Mammon, the very embodiment of corrosive Greed. Mammon personified that single vice, a bit like his master Satan, who, at least since his name was borrowed from the Babylonians, has embodied evil of every kind.

Some decades after that odd birth, the newborn infant, grown up and become a vagabond preacher, nailed down a contradiction: "You can't serve both God and Mammon; it won't work. One of them will win out." And his life was that of a committed anti-Mammonite. He and his ragtag followers hiked from village to village without even a change of clothes, buying a little food, when they needed it, from a common purse.

Frequently they had no roof to sleep under, much less a bed. As the vagabond once said, "Foxes have their dens and birds their nests, but the Son of Man has nowhere to lay his head." In fact, most nights under a roof he spent on a dirt floor, and his bent elbow was his only pillow. But by day he preached on, denouncing Mammon, and promoting selfless love.

When this man came to a bad end, as so often happens to those who challenge comforting vice, his executioners threw dice for this pauper's only possession of value: his tunic, simple but seamlessly made by his mother. (We don't know who won it, but he went home happy. Another possession, you see.) Many would say the story ended then, with Mammon winning. Christians don't.

Mammon did win many centuries later, in a steadily wealthier America, one dominated by material values relentlessly pounded into it by the media advertising. And Christmas, that celebrated the vagabond's birth? Well, the shallow, mammonized culture held onto the sentimental elements of the story, swaddling them in carols that, these days, are outplayed by the other ones about Frosty and Rudolf. Oh, and ones about that ersatz god in red flannel and fake fur—you know, the one who "sees you when you're sleeping, knows when you're awake."

Over the years, preparation for the old holyday became a frenzy of searching and spending, hauling and wrapping, acid reflux, sore feet, and thumping headaches. And the day itself was lost in a snowstorm of torn gift wrap and in an orgy of food and drink. If the day goes well, children and adults crawl into bed drunk with gifts, sated, stupefied as zombies. Mammon surely smiles on them in their restless sleep. For, except for churchgoing that some managed to work in, it's been his kind of day, start to finish.

Until this year, which may show that Mammon overplayed his hand. He has so successfully drugged the wealthy and powerful with Greed that he over-tipped the economy

that feeds Greed among us lesser humans. With the economy suddenly, crazily out of control, we are now scared to
spend. Everybody's cutting back except, evidently, those
buying for their kids. A mother on TV last week said pi-
ously that she and her husband weren't buying much for
each other this year. "But I'd never short-change my kids,"
she added proudly.

Right, mom. Trade away a good chance to talk to the
kids about the world's state and the whole family's need to
tighten their belts. Instead, reinforce the words of a current
ad. It features scores of baritones chanting, "I want it all! I
want it all! And I want it NOW!" A Mammon-inspired
hymn, that one.

But among those old carols, the ones elbowed off the
airwaves by ballads about reindeer and snowmen, there is
one that still embodies what that long-ago birth was about.
Set aside the usual melody, please. It's too saccharine, unworthy of the profound lyrics. Just think about the words of
its first verse.

They address Bethlehem, that little town of crowds and
dusty streets. Now the town is silent, dreamlessly asleep under the canopy of distant gleaming stars. But something is at
work in you, Bethlehem, says the song. And then the line
that tells the whole story: "The hopes and fears of all the
years are met in thee tonight."

The fears of all ages, past and to come, that there won't
be money enough, or food or clothing or shelter or safety.
Or that we won't get everything we want before we die.
That we won't die.

The hopes? That something, someone, will reach into
our midst to make everything right; straighten us out, in
spite of ourselves.

"The hopes and fears" of that hymn are what that odd
birth was all about. And the vagabond preacher's life and
sublime teaching. And his horrible death and his triumph.

Back in ancient Bethlehem, an intervention into the dysfunctional human family! Now, that's worth singing about. That's worth celebrating.

Harrowing Times at Heathrow

Anne and I just came back from three weeks in England. That's a trip I never expected to make again. But my other companion Parkinson, as whimsical as he is relentless, took a vacation himself a couple of months ago. (I'll explain the likely causes in another column.) I was left free, at least temporarily, from some of the worst symptoms. And so my bride and I decided, quite suddenly, that we'd run under the silent guns and make the trip.

It was wonderful, especially since friends conspired to pass us along, one to another, making travel easy for me. We drove to Boston, left the car with good friends, and were driven to Logan Airport. Since I'm poorly equipped now to stand in lines, we'd phoned ahead for disabled assistance, and a wheelchair driver met us at the door. This man whisked us around the lines, right up to luggage check-in. Then, with our carry-ons piled on top of me, he steered right up to the security gate, put our chattel onto the scanner for us, and braced the chair and me as I stood to walk through the metal detector. Then we were zoomed on to a waiting area.

We needed to wait because, following the airline's standard directions, we had arrived three hours early—for a process that had taken only about twenty minutes. But, no complaints. That disabled assistance sure was a tremendous blessing, going and coming back, and despite an unplanned adventure when we got to London Heathrow.

As we left the plane, the stewardess told us to climb the ramp and be seated; another wheelchair would soon arrive.

And indeed, one did, this time pushed by a big smiling Caribbean with not much command of English. I got loaded up, again piled with the two backpacks and my sleep-apnea gear in its own box, and we wheeled off toward passport control. I had only to ride and, of course, hold the load in place with both hands and my chin.

It was a long run, and halfway Anne got to step onto a moving walkway as we wheeled along beside her. That's where the adventure began. From far down the long corridor, high-balling along towards me, came an empty wheelchair pushed by a short, rather broad woman. She was calling out in what may have been Turkish, and she had fire in her eye. I thought for a moment she was going to ram us. My own wheeler stopped short, and my Anne was carried away by the moving walkway.

The squarish woman didn't ram us but squealed to a stop, blocking our way. Then she went at it, hammer and tongs, at the Caribbean twice her height. Hers, it turned out, was our assigned wheelchair, and the amiable Caribbean was a gypsy driver who'd pirated her passenger, and hence her tip.

She won. I was bustled out of his chair and into hers, the carry-ons were re-piled on top of me, and we sped off, the woman still muttering imprecations at the gypsy. We caught up with Anne and hustled on toward passport check. But, almost there, I heard a loud clank. The right footrest had fallen off the chair.

"Bad equipment!" she shouted in English. "Very bad equipment." It sounded like a phrase she'd had many occasions to use. Suddenly she was squatting next to the chair, pounding the footrest on the terrazzo floor.

"Quiet!" Anne pleaded. "My husband has trouble with startle reflex!" (And, like many fellow Parkies, I do—if I don't foresee the cause of a loud noise. This time, I did: a squarish woman squatting, slamming a shaft of metal on the floor.) But she quickly got it fixed, reinstalled it, and soon was rushing us along again, up to and through the passport check.

Customs and luggage were down one floor, so Anne stepped onto a very long escalator while the squarish woman and I headed for the top of a pair of long ramps. She was still muttering, "Bad equipment!" as we got to the first ramp, but then she switched her complaint. "No brakes!"

Well. Since we've been home, I've watched a lot of Olympic ski-jumping. Every time skiers throw themselves down that awful first drop, I relive my Heathrow ramp experience. Indeed, there were no brakes on the chair, and I plunged down that thirty-degree slope with only the woman's sheer strength holding us both back. I couldn't look back, but I'm sure she left a parallel trail of smoking rubber from her shoe heels.

"Bad equipment!" she shouted as we made a sharp turn and were briefly on a level stretch. "No brakes!" and we hurtled down the second ramp.

Anne, on the escalator, missed the whole adventure; and you can see that I lived through it. Shaken but laughing in spite of myself, I was wheeled to luggage pick-up and then through a perfunctory customs check. Breathless, we found ourselves in the crowded airport lobby.

The squarish lady seemed to have bonded with us. She was suddenly maternal and reluctant to leave us. But we insisted we were fine, and we sent her off with a hefty tip that was partly a bribe. When she wheeled away, we felt relieved and released.

I've since had leisure to wonder: Had she played out that whole scenario repeatedly and found it always worked? Did she end up splitting the tip with the Caribbean?

Working Along the Border

Lately I've been back in the company of undertakers, lots of them. You may remember that last summer I attended the annual convention of the New York State Funeral Directors Association. This was at the invitation of Gordon Terry of Edmeston, who had just been elected president of that very large group.

Gordon invited Anne and me to attend the convention with him and his wife Joan so that I could serve as the president's chaplain. The office wasn't overloaded with convention responsibilities. I gave an invocation, presided over a moving memorial service for deceased colleagues, and gave a continuing education lecture titled, "And Survived by her Husband ..." The lecture dealt with men's grieving and how different, and often less effective, it is from women's.

The lecture went well, and last month Gordon invited me to repeat it, this time for the funeral directors of this part of the state. I now faced a smaller audience of about fifty this time, but it was just as attentive, just as ready to add comments. But let me tell you more about last summer's experience.

The men and women in the big auditorium listened closely and often nodded when I touched something in their own professional experience. For instance, I noted the difference in openness of grieving among men of southern European stock and those of English, Celtic, or northern European heritage. That caused lots of heads to nod and brought wonderful revelations for me in the question-and-comment period.

For where I had talked about those differences expressed on the funeral director's couch, as a family sat around the father and planned the mother's service, the men and women at the convention spoke most movingly about an earlier stage, when they and their staff arrived at the home after the death. They spoke feelingly about the variations of widowers' reactions that greeted them, from grief vented in sobs, tears, even groans, to men who stood flattened against a bedroom wall, their faces stony masks sometimes scarlet from trying to suppress shameful, unmanly tears.

Several directors spoke of the need to let the family take charge in that bedroom, and told of his personal outrage when his own father died in Florida. When the local undertaker arrived, he immediately ordered the family out of the room. The son, an undertaker himself, protested and was told that the law required them to leave.

"The hell it does!" he shouted, grief giving way to rage. And he ordered the interloper and his crew into another room until the family had prepared the old man themselves, washing his body lovingly, dressing it in fresh pajamas, lifting it onto the gurney and even carrying it downstairs to the van. "Now's your time," he said to his tight-lipped colleague.

"Ever since then," he said, "the first thing I ask on arriving at a home is, "Have you spent enough time saying goodbye?" and "Shall we wait in the living room while you tend to your loved one?" Those questions, he told us, can help numbing shock give place to a sense of control and to real grieving.

He sat down but then stood up again. "And something else I've learned: If you're finishing the arrangements at the house and have had the family place their loved one in a body bag, never, NEVER zip up that bag in their presence. That sound can also throw them right back into a shocked sense that something is being ripped from their lives and is being carried away. And the sound will stay in their memories forever."

A woman director then stood to back him up. "Look," she said, "our business is not to serve the dead. They are already on their way, beyond any help we can give them. It's the living that we serve. And everything we do should give them strength and stability in a time when their lives have been knocked out of focus." And again, heads nodded all around that big room. I even heard an "Amen."

Oh, wow. What a piece of continuing education that comment period was for me! And what a time of soaring admiration for these men and women who work along the border between life and death, who help us negotiate unfamiliar and frightening terrain.

I've several treasured friends who are funeral directors; Gordon and Joan, of course, but also Cooperstown's own Martin Tillapaugh and Peter Deysenroth. I've long known their deep humaneness; but since I often preside at funerals, I've also watched with admiration, even awe, as they quietly do their most fundamental job: helping grievers, people half stunned by loss, through the worst of times.

Our life's path runs parallel to the border on which these men and women work. The border is within sight, out of the corner of our eye; we studiously avoid glancing that way. But the time comes, as it must in each of our lives, when we must approach that border with a loved one. It's comforting to know that help awaits us there.

Back to Baltimore

We went to Baltimore again for a second consultancy with Dr. Zoltan Mari of the Johns Hopkins Parkinson's clinic. I liked Dr. Mari on sight when we met him last year: a big, tousled Hungarian with a warm smile and laser eyes. I love his first name and think his stationery should have a logo in the upper left corner, a dramatic lightning bolt right next to "Zoltan."

Before we saw Dr. Mari this time, we had a half hour with an equally pleasant resident named Dr. Valeriy Parfenov. Valeriy, who had a faint Slavic accent, took all the usual vitals and asked the standard questions, but then echoed some of Dr. Mari's tests of last year. He tapped joints of legs and arms with a rubber mallet, then touched a tuning fork to various spots to see if I could feel the vibration, then had me walk down a corridor and back while he watched my gait.

All this and more Valeriy did with a friendly professionalism that gave him high marks in my book. Then, with a smile and raised eyebrows, he said, "I go to show my notes to the big boss. We'll be back soon."

Fifteen minutes later he was back, following the "big boss" into the room. Dr. Mari shook Anne's and my hands, greeted us by name, and settled into a chair next to us. Valeriy stood respectfully just behind him, taking notes. There followed a leisured half hour of close questioning, plus Dr. Mari's own tests of my vitals and reflexes. As we talked, he referenced Dr. Deringer's notes since last year, and the psycho-neurological report done by Dr. Connie Jones at Bassett.

"She gave you exactly the right tests, all of them," he said, running a finger down the long list. He looked up and grinned.

"She also says you're a smart guy." Then we talked about the tests' basic finding: My verbal skills are still pretty much intact, but my capacities for analysis and abstract thought have eroded, and my short-term memory, too.

That's just the way it feels from inside me, I told him. He nodded and asked for examples. Anne and I had plenty of them.

At the end, Dr. Mari said my symptoms have intensified since last year, but still not enough to nail down a diagnosis more precise than "Parkinsonism." Still more maturing of symptoms is required. I reminded him that he'd said that he could give an instant diagnosis from an autopsy. (Behind him, Valeriy broke into a broad grin, as if to say, "That sounds like the old man!") But Dr. Mari, after pretending a moment's consideration, said that autopsy was still too extreme a measure.

He did say that what would be a big help was one or another of two rare and high-priced scans, neither of them covered by insurance. "What we need to find," he said, "is a research program making use of one of the tests." He'd gladly recommend my admission and would start looking for one.

That was good news, even though most of the rest wasn't too heartening. I'm losing ground to a still-unspecified disease that is compromising, not only my bodily functions, but also my brain. Please pray or cross your fingers, as is your wont, that we turn up a source for those tests—and that they're being offered in Buffalo, not Budapest.

In Transit

It may have been the most fully packed ten-minute span of my life, containing two adventures I'm not likely to forget. The adventures are notably different, and yet their meanings do merge.

Some months ago, Anne and I were traveling on Interstate 81, heading for a visit to Johns Hopkins. Blue was traveling with us; he stayed with dog-friendly friends down there while we saw the Hopkins docs.

Somewhere well into the seven-hour drive, we decided to pull into one of the indistinguishable rest stops. Blue, you see, probably needed to stretch his four legs and raise one a few times. In the parking lot, we decided that Anne would escort Blue to the doggie walk and return with him to the car in ten minutes. By that time I was to visit the gent's room myself, then return to the car so that Anne could go inside. And so I headed for the building, with no hint of the events that lay just ahead.

But not in the men's room. In there, stolid men stood at the urinals, gazing straight ahead. Almost all of them also observed the men's room protocol of total silence, even the ones splashing water as they washed up at the sinks. The one exception was a forty-something who was managing (can you believe it?) simultaneously to void and talk on his cell phone. His tone was endearing, but I wonder what his sweetheart made of the echoing sounds of flushing.

I was back out in the lobby quickly, with lots of my ten minutes to give over to loitering and watching. The place was packed, with long lines of exhausted parents and cranky or manic kids in front of McDonald's, TCBY, and Auntie Anne's Pretzels. The manic kids who could break away were galloping around between the lines and among the people crowding in and out of the lobby. Dead center in the lobby, in the very best spot to impede traffic, a domestic crisis started that soon drew the attention of the manic tots, and mine, too.

A little blonde of about three had been refused something by her dad, who stood stoically while the little girl, who'd failed with whining and wheedling, shifted to tragic tears, then to stamping and blubbering. The father remained unmoved, and so she fell back on a three-year old girl's ultimate weapon. She squatted like a plaster garden gnome, filled her lungs to absolute capacity, and began to shriek like rent metal.

You know the sound I mean. It seems impossibly loud from such a small source; but there it is, the equivalent in intensity to a surgical laser beam, not only tearing at your eardrums but somehow also piercing right between your eyebrows.

The shriek was not only agonizingly loud, but endless. That tot never broke for breath and must have been drawing air in through her ears. And the place where she squatted was also perfect for sending the shriek up among the rafters and back down on everyone. (It surely echoed inside the men's room, and I'm guessing that some of the startled men standing in there briefly lost their streams.) In the lobby, the milling hundreds had mostly turned toward the tot, some with hands over their ears; and a lot of those manic kids now stood near her, admiring her technique.

I can't do justice to the paralyzing intensity of that shriek; to hear its match, you'd have to visit some place fabricating steel. In minutes more, bulbs would have been popping overhead and the plastic letters and numbers would have been raining off the McDonald's menu signs.

But finally the scarlet-faced dad gave up and tried to lift

his daughter to her feet. She, however, had locked herself in that gnome-like squat. In desperation, dad swept her up and under his arm like a bundle of kindling and carried her, still shrieking, toward the doors. People backed away to clear a path.

The first pair of doors closed behind her, but we could still hear her. The second closed, and we still could, even as the dad strode away across the parking lots. I'm guessing that by then dogs were howling on neighboring farms and cows bellowing out in the fields.

Inside, folks took awhile to adjust to the relative quiet, but soon things were back to normal, with manic kids careening again among the travel-worn adults.

Meanwhile, with time still to spare, I stood with ringing ears, thinking about that outraged, primal shriek. Forgive me, but she'd offered a metaphor for most human lives. The little blonde had voiced the essence of a child's morality —the morality that, if we're not careful, is ours for all of our days.

A child's moral code says, "Good is what I want, evil is anything that blocks me from it." Until corrected, the child's code has no place for consequences, no place for rights of anyone, or anything, outside of self. That egoist's code is poignantly embodied in the Eden temptation story, and it has since been called "original sin." Maybe it might better be called the "originating sin," for every type in evil's catalog is merely a variation, a continuation of childish, irresponsible selfishness.

Individuals practice it, as do groups, as do nations, as does the whole human race. It's in us as toddlers and, un-checked, it will be with us throughout life and to the grave. We'll die, our souls still screeching something comparable to the little tot's "I WANT WHAT I WANT!"

The young girl's was a bravura performance, and a great illustration of a trait that, sadly, many of us adults, "children of a larger growth," carry through life and to the grave. For many humans, almost every choice, big and small, echoes the essence of the toddler's shriek, "I WANT WHAT I WANT!" It makes for much personal unhappiness.

Great minds out of the East have said that all pain is caused by desire, and the work of our lifetimes is quietly to subdue and reduce desire. Maybe they're on to something.

The second adventure began after the little girl was gone and the lobby had settled to its' normal buzzing swirl of people, I still had some time left to loiter and watch. (I was awaiting, you may remember, Anne's arrival from walking Blue, my signal to go out and sit with Blue in the car.) And so I stood to the side and out of the way, against a blank wall just past Auntie Anne's Pretzels.

There were lots of careworn adults to watch, and cranky kids, too, though none to match that little screecher. I watched one weary family group—mother, father, daughter, son—standing in the McDonald's line, endearingly leaning against each other. I saw an old gent scuff slowly toward a marble column, bump his forehead against it and stop, maybe to enjoy its cool surface, maybe because he just hadn't seen it in his path.

But across that crowded lobby, through the moving skein of bodies big and small, I saw something arresting and beautiful. And there began my second adventure in ten minutes. In fact, it only took three minutes, but I doubt that I'll ever forget it.

Standing against the opposite wall was a man about my height and age, but he was not loitering and watching. He was motionless, and his dark eyes were slightly raised above the crowd scene. His rich mahogany-toned skin and classic features identified him as a Dravidian from southernmost India. And so did his dress, all of it a brilliant white.

His snowy tunic almost reached his knees; beneath it he wore loose white trousers. Around his shoulders was a scarf, wide and full, and again it almost reached his knees. Above his dark face and full gray beard and mustache, he wore a white turban wound from soft, snowy gauze. Unwound, the strip must have been ten feet long.

My eyes were riveted on him, this figure of total composure beyond the swirling crowd of people. And, though this is difficult to describe, something deep in me began to respond. Across the crowd, I felt linked to him, drawn to him. And I began to walk toward him, through the crowds.

When I was halfway across the lobby, his eyes met mine and a wondrous smile broke out on his face. I raised my hands, palms together, up to my chin in *namaste*, the Indian greeting. He did the same, still smiling, but with a luminous softness now in his features.

Namaste, you may know, isn't a simple "hello." In its origin, it means, "That of God in me greets that of God in you."

As I approached, this grand man began to chuckle, and he spread his arms. The hug he then gave me was the sort one gives on suddenly meeting an old friend. Then he took me by the elbows; I did the same, and we stood smiling at each other. Not knowing whether he spoke English, I gestured with my head to the lobby's other side and said slowly, "I felt light coming from you."

His head tipped back in another joyful chuckle. And then he raised his right hand and placed the heel of his palm high on my forehead, fingertips resting on what's left of my hair. The few Hindi words he murmured were surely a blessing.

Then, this smiling, gentle man nodded slowly at me, and I back at him. And I walked away, down the swarming lobby. And here came Anne, just walking in the doors at the far end.

I didn't look back, almost fearful the man would have disappeared. But he would have still been there. He was no apparition; he was as real as I am. But his blessing changed me. These days when I praise my Creator through Jesus, I no longer center myself behind my closed eyes. My consciousness drifts in the darkness up to my forehead, where I still sense the soft pressure of that hand.

Oh, friends, we cannot cage such a Being of Infinite Love inside a rigid palisade of dogma. Grace is everywhere, everywhere.

Arm-in-Arm

When I was first diagnosed with Parkinson's three years ago, Anne and I felt knocked to our knees. But at once she said firmly, "You must write about this in your column. Others out there are suffering from it." And so I began the series of columns that are the backbone of this book and that, if God intends, will continue in the paper beyond your reading of the book.

Within days of the first column, I began getting phone calls, mostly from women whose husbands had Parkinson's, but sometimes from the men themselves. With the latter, the tone was always relief that, thank God, someone was talking about what they were experiencing. They were suddenly not alone.

When, with the help of two healthcare professionals, we had organized ourselves into a support group, I approached the first meeting with some real misgivings. Did I really want to meet with men who probably already embodied what was to be my future?

It turned out that that fear was in every one of us as we gathered, walking awkwardly, leaning on canes and on walkers, even trundling in wheelchairs. But the fear disappeared as soon as we began to talk. It was replaced with relief and literal exclamations of, "You, too?" Suddenly each of us had company besides Parkinson's itself.

And relief was just as profound for the care-partners. They were all women since initially we thought that the group must be all men; we'd thought that we would feel too awkward talking about some of the personal problems that

Parkinson's brings—plumbing problems, for instance. (We are well past that concern now and are about to welcome our first women Parkies.)

The women care-partners had almost all been closeted in their own homes by their husband's sickness. Now, suddenly, they were spending an hour out in the world with their husbands, and then—hallelujah!—an hour in company with other women dealing with the same challenges. Talk about win-win!

Unlike some other support groups, which might better be called "information groups," our sessions were mutual sharing from the first meeting. We talked about everything related to our experiences with the disease—imbalance, sexual frustration, freezing as we walked or climbed stairs.

And most of all we admitted fear of public embarrassment from shaking or grimacing, shaking or splashing coffee on ourselves or others. Men, we all acknowledged, are creatures of fragile ego; whence the temptation to say "Screw it!" and just hide at home, incurring guilt from paralyzing a loved spouse's life. What venting! What relief, and so often comic!

We did have invited speakers: speech and physical therapists, dieticians, neurologists, social service personnel. But the focus remained on own our sharing and coping. And it still does.

Perhaps two examples will show just how the support group has not only bolstered individuals, but fused us into a band of tottering brothers. The first concerns our senior member, a bright, incisive retired medical man that I'll call Ken.

Ken was well into a Parkinsonism subset called Lewey Body Syndrome. Speech therapy that, early on, might have given him a new hold on speaking had not taken place. Consequently Ken's voice had sunken to a slurred whisper.

One afternoon, after the care-partners had left for their separate meeting, we guys were sitting around the coffee and cake they'd so thoughtfully left for us. A member of the group said idly, "Ken, can you still shout?" Ken gave a snort and shook his head. But the other man, remembering a lesson from his own speech therapy, wouldn't let go.

"Hey," he said, "here's an experiment. I've been to your house and looked out the patio door at that beautiful lawn and shrubbery and back fence." (I'd seen that fence, too: six feet tall and painted a pristine white.)

"OK, imagine you're looking out there and see a teenager with an aerosol can. He's about to paint graffiti on that fence. You go to the door and you bellow at him!

And then the man bellowed, "HEY, YOU LITTLE BASTARD! GET THE HELL AWAY FROM THAT FENCE!"

Everyone laughed, but then Ken drew a deep, crackling breath, and yelled, "HEY, YOU LITTLE BASTARD! GET AWAY FROM MY FENCE!"

That brought cheers, and Ken actually grinned. But then he composed himself and spoke—ten decibels louder than usual. "I normally don't use such language," he said reprovingly. That drew more laughter that he obviously enjoyed.

The second illustration also took place over coffee and cake. We'd been trading notes on our past employments. Knowing he had a doctorate in physics, I queried another member. "Burt, did you teach physics in some college?"

Burt, like most in the group, sometimes had a memory freeze when he could not pull forward even the most significant elements of his past. I watched his face contort with effort, but nothing would come. Then, as we watched in silent awe, his right hand rose and scribed a perfect circle at arm's length in front of him. Burt then muttered a single word: "Greenbelt."

Well, back in my days as a monk, I lived for nearly ten years near Greenbelt, Maryland. The National Agricultural Research Center is there, but that graceful arc suggested to me another place, just down the road.

"Burt, were you at Goddard Space Center?" At those words, Burt broke into a radiant smile and began to talk, slowly and clearly.

Our Burt, so modest a presence among us, had been a young Naval Officer on the mission staff at Goddard, early in the US space program. Our physicist Burt had painstakingly planned the crucial orbits that assured safety, indeed survival, of astronauts on the early missions. It was Burt who had agonized to match calculations of minutes and seconds against supersonic speed, against available fuel, against his wondrous curving trajectories; all to guarantee safe departure, rendezvous, re-entry, and safe landing.

Our friend had been an absolutely critical figure in all of that; and in our meeting as the memory flooded back into his consciousness, Burt smiled in relief and a sense of quiet pride. What a fine moment for him, for all of us.

Playwright Tennessee Williams, who was painfully estranged from his fellow humans, once skewered himself with this wry comment: "If so many are lonely as seem to be lonely, it would be inexcusably selfish to be alone."

Right on, Tennessee, and God rest you! We Parkies up here in Central New York State have taken you at your word. We're past being lonely alone. Laughing at ourselves, we're stumbling along, arm in arm.

When Cows Go Bad

I don't know where they'll be when you read this, but right now a gang of renegade heifers is at large in Fly Creek. For over a week they've been roving around a couple of square miles. Locals announce sightings as if they were yetis: "Saw 'em Tuesday way down by The Cornfields!" "They were along Allison Road yesterday, grazing with five big deer." "Hey, Bill Preston was standing on his deck, turned around, and his yard was full of cows!"

They're only seven in number, but they're big—about nine hundred pounds each. And one heifer is enormously pregnant. Shame on her, joining that pack of runaways! Dr. Phil would have something to say to her, I'll bet.

I can't be sure, but probably that bulging heifer now dearly wants to be back in Gerry Day's fenced pasture, secure and well fed. When Anne and I spotted her on the past Sunday, she was standing with the other runaways in our big hayfield, looking miserable. The whole time we watched, Mattie (not her real name) never joined the others in grazing on the new grass. Instead she just stood, head down, her back legs splayed to support an udder swollen with milk and bigger than a bushel basket.

Beside being really uncomfortable, she must be confused, too. Nobody explained to Mattie what is happening to her—certainly not that damned bull. She's been feeling poorly for weeks, and now sudden twists and bumps occur deep inside her. And with every step, that huge bag, stretched and prickly, almost knocks her off her hoofs. Each bit of stubble that pokes it makes her wince.

No question, Mattie should never have gotten in with that high-kicking crowd. But they had all been excited that day, mooing and milling around. Linda and John Kosmer, who are building a home up on Day Road, believe they know what started the ruckus. They're having a well drilled, and they think that the machine's steady, heavy thumping spooked the heifers.

Maybe so. Or maybe boredom or high spirits sent them over that low spot in the fence. I imagine Mattie hanging back uncertainly as the others cleared the wire like cows jumping over the moon. But then Mattie made her own move, abruptly following the crowd. (We're never more herd animals than when we're teens, right? And, after all, you're only a heifer once.)

Whatever the cause, out they all went, first onto the gravel of Day Road, then, giddy with freedom, into the mowed hayfield on the other side. But that wasn't enough. Some troublemaker among them took charge and led them through that field, into the Senifs' yard, then onto the edge of Route 26. That's where my startled wife saw them. She pulled up short as they started across the roadway to disappear into the tall corn. That was Friday, August 18, the day of the breakout.

When Anne got home she phoned the Days at once. But of course it was too late. By the time Gerry could get there, that bunch of excited teens was deep into the cornfield near The Cornfields (a grand old social club that belongs to the Slovenian Benevolent Society). Acres of tall stalks there made a great hiding place. Gerry tried to rout them out, as did his wife and his son and assorted friends. But no luck.

A cow breakout was the last thing Gerry needed. A hard-working dairy farmer, he'd just finished an especially hard, rainy haying time. With all the cutting, baling, loading, hauling, and stowing thousands of bales finally done, Gerry had started to settle back to his ordinary level of grinding work. That has him up before light to hook forty-four cows to the milking machines. Next comes a morning of sterilizing the equipment, then cleaning stalls, feeding, shifting stock from field to field, till it's time for evening milking. Then more sterilizing. That's Gerry's life, seven days a week.

Having the heifers in his field up on Day Road, away from the dairy herd, made things a little easier—or did, till one found that low spot in the fence. Now Gerry and his family are losing part of each day to fruitless searches. On Sunday the 20th, Anne and I got caught up in the quest.

We were in the kitchen when I glanced out front to see men across the road, looking anxiously our way and waving their arms. "Are we on fire?" I thought, and headed out the back door to check. I got no farther than the porch when, just outside the screening, a cavalcade of heifers clomped up the driveway. They headed through our backyard, the waving men following.

The more people you have to herd loose cows, the better; and so Anne and I joined the wavers as they drove them down our other driveway and swung them left on Allison Road. The heifers' turn was too broad, and they tromped through our neighbor's side yard before heading down Allison, toward the bridge.

Now we're on track, I thought. If we get them across the bridge and swing them left, they're on their way to Gerry's farm and captivity again. But, as Arrie Hecox used to say, "Cows hate bridges!" These heifers, true to form, caught sight of the bridge and suddenly veered left, across the Prestons' lawn, and crashed into our woods along Oaks Creek.

It wasn't hard to follow their wide trail through the shady woods. It led about a quarter mile and then broke into the sunlight again—at the back of our big hayfield on Allison Road.

Now was the time to try swinging them back toward Day Road, where the whole mess started. But no. Those flighty heifers wheeled and headed southwest, forded Fly Creek, and disappeared into the tall corn again. My heart ached for Gerry as he stood, slowly shaking his head.

Keep a watch for those heifers, please. Call Gerry, especially if you see them trekking toward Milford or lined up to board a bus for somewhere. Those girls all need to come back home. Especially Mattie.

Strangers on a Train

Carol Holmes, a Quaker friend down in New York City, emailed me a video-clip I wish I could show to each of you. The best I can do, however, is to describe it. The title is "Bodhisattva on the Metro."

The Metro is the Paris subway system, and all action takes place inside one of its cars. The Buddhist *bodhisattva* is, in this case, a man who has so purified himself that he ought to have been freed from *samsara,* the burden of rebirth. But this man so loves his fellow humans that he's chosen to stay on in this lifetime. He aims to help others to discover that all suffering is rooted in desire for physical or even spiritual things, but that desire itself can be quelled by a life of simplicity, quiet detachment, meditation, and selfless love of others. (It's a gentle faith, Buddhism, in spite of those who shed blood in its name.)

This *bodhisattva* carries out his ministry to others on the Metro. The train car he enters is full of people with frowns, scowls, tense faces, or glazed eyes. Some are trying to sleep, their heads against the windows. Others try reading newspapers or magazines or books. Some look weary, and others dead-tired. There is, of course, no interaction among them. Each sits or slumps in isolation.

The *bodhisattva* sits down next to a black woman whose face is a tragic mask; she looks lost in rehearsing a litany of personal woes. Her new companion sits quietly as the train begins to move, but then a smile begins to flicker on his broad face.

The smile is soon a grin, like that of someone recalling a

very funny story. His features begin to crinkle, his eyes widen as if he were suppressing laughter. Then a snort escapes his nose, and he begins to laugh softly, then more loudly. People around him frown, and then turn slightly toward him reprovingly. But now his laughter is full-blown, his face is wreathed in merriment, he gasps for breath between outbursts.

As each outburst comes, the other riders begin to glance toward one another, as if to share their disapproval of this madman. But then one, shaking his head, begins himself to chuckle. Others smile, snort, and break into laughter. Newspapers and books are closed as hilarity sweeps through the car. Soon people are whooping, leaning on one another's shoulders. And every time the general laughter pauses, another laugh from the pleasant little round-faced man sets them all off again.

The collection of strangers has become a community of joy, shared and out of control. But as the car pulls into a station, they all try to sober themselves, as children do when a teacher reenters the classroom.

Then a staid, tall old man in business dress steps onto the car and pauses, rolled umbrella against his chest, surveying the group sternly. That does it. The whole lot bursts into unchecked laughter, rocking in their seats, tears running down some cheeks. The staid old man recoils, then walks quickly to the far end of the car, away from these fools. That, of course, convulses them even more. They're sure that the old man thinks that he's stepped into a lunatic ward. More whoops, roars, gasps.

Then comes the end of the line, and all the laughers begin to file off, some leaning against others, wiping their eyes, all gulping and panting from laughing for so long and so hard. They squeeze one another's arms, pat each other's backs. And then they walk off into separate worlds.

As the last leaves the car, the camera peers in to where the *bodhisattva* had sat. He's not there, but then we spot him through the far window, in a crowded train on the adjoining track. That train begins to move, and the little man begins to smile, then grin. The train disappears down the track, but we know exactly what's going on inside.

And has anything changed in the lives of those others, now walking down sidewalks to climb stairs and unlock doors? I'm guessing that, as they walk, they chuckle as often as they think back on their madcap, carefree happiness. They even laugh out loud, making passersby turn and stare. I'm guessing that, as days and weeks pass, they'll still be recalling that touchstone event with wonder.

And, when riding the Metro daily, should one of them see a companion from that time of uncapped, zany joy, they'll smile warmly and knowingly, as if they share a secret of some sort. Neither can name the secret, but that doesn't matter a bit.

In the Winter Darkness

Lovers of dogs and cats reading the following will understand at once. Another reaction will come from those who just don't understand pets: "Well, you fools! It serves you right!"

I'm bunking down these days in my study to give Anne respite from my Parkinson's restlessness. It is a great arrangement, with her right across the hall in a welcoming queen-sized bed and with a new TV. And I have a comfortable single bed in what I now think of as my "man cave." My bed, desk, books, lounger, laptop—what more could I ask? And most nights I have the company of Simon the cat. It's like camping out for us guys!

Simon spends many nights at the bottom of the bed, right between my ankles. But cat lovers will understand he also likes to settle on some high eminence in the room. His favorite spot in the man cave is atop the Xerox copier. It's suitably high and placed just next to the west window. Hunkered there, Simon has a view across the west field and right down Allison Road, almost to the bridge.

I've put a thick throw of rough-woven wool on the machine's top and know he's grateful for it in his catlike way. Which is to say, he recognizes its value and is glad that I know what is due to him. I find that an endearing quality in cats. Others may call me wacko.

One recent night, Simon was enthroned on the Xerox and I was deeply asleep, settled down for a long winter's nap. Sometime in the small hours, I half awoke to a low electrical growl and then a couple of clicks, but then sank right back into sleep. A minute later, or maybe an hour, I came awake again to "thunk, thunk, whirrr," and again, "thunk, thunk, whirr."

The Xerox was running. Simon was over there, making copies.

I jumped up and cut him off after three sheets. On his part, he rolled over and stretched, then meowed inquiringly. I guess that, shifting earlier in his sleep, he had pushed the machine's "ON" button. Then, later, he'd hit "PRINT." Repeatedly.

OK, no fault, no penalty. Except to my sleep. For it took awhile for me to settle down again. After all, what to my wondering eyes had appeared? A gray-and-white cat, printing copies in the night. If I had any dreams after that, I'll bet they were interesting ones. Sheep at electronic pianos, maybe, and hens lined up like Rockettes, kicking up drumsticks high in front of them.

The only disadvantage of my man cave is that it's right above the kitchen, and that's where Blue the dog sleeps. And does so soundly, unless internal distress makes him think, "I gotta go—right now!" When that happens, he begins moaning, at first softly to himself.

If conditions worsen, he shifts to a low register and begins sounding like Long John Silver. "Arrrr," he says, and then, "Arrrr!" But there's also a whiny, background wheeze, as if the crusty old pirate were choking on a fish bone.

All this I can hear through the floor and am intended to. And when I get up, pulling my feet from under a disturbed Simon, I sometimes open the bedroom door to find Blue standing right there, dancing from foot to foot, all wriggles and smiles and wagging tail.

He knows he has violated a major house rule: "THOU SHALT NOT, OH DOG, PAD FROM KITCHEN INTO DINING ROOM, MUCH LESS UP THE STAIRS, LEST THY TAIL BE SHOVED UP THY BUTT AND SNATCHED OUT THROUGH THY JAWS, TURNING

THEE <u>INSIDE OUT</u>!" But all his dancing and smiling is to convince me that desperation has trumped the ordinary rules. I, of course, buy it.

Downstairs we go. I add to my bathrobe my outdoor coat and my red Elmer Fudd cap, and we head out into the Arctic darkness. I have him on a leash and am almost jerked after him as he streaks for a favorite unloading depot. I stand shivering, admiring Orion overhead lying at rest on his back, as I'd sooner be. But then Blue gallops back in a kind of victory run, and back we go into the house's warmth.

There's a reason I have Blue on a leash during such night treks. There have been several of them lately, all following of a single cause. Somewhere down in our woods is something in a horrible state of decay. Blue is ecstatic over it, and keeps running off to fetch home more pieces. So we keep him under protective arrest. It's protective for us, for what he hauls home is beyond description.

Somehow he got away from Anne a few nights ago and galloped off into the woods. My Anne, single-minded in her devotion, ran off after him. And, as darkness deepened, her wobbly husband trundled after both of them. I caught up with Anne at the far end of the property, halfway down a steep, snow-covered slope.

"Get back to the house!" she yelled, "You'll fall down!" This from a dear woman of a certain age, in the blackness and halfway down a snowy slope, with every chance of snagging her foot in brambles and tumbling all the way down and into Oaks Creek.

Then I heard a distant woof.

"He's back up by the house!" I shouted and headed that way. Sure enough, there stood Blue, just outside the sheep gate. Whatever he had dragged back from the woods, he had already hidden for future reference.

Everybody got back inside safely, but on toward morning I heard the choking pirate below me again. And so I unsettled Simon, opened the bedroom door, and found that dancing, apologetic dog.

Why put up with such things? For petless people, I have no answer. For others, none is needed.

Yoked as One

Unless one lives reclusive and unloved, the yoke of Parkinsonism isn't borne alone. Others near us share it through compassion and help. Most usually a single other person becomes what the literature calls "primary caregiver," or "care-partner." These two, patient and partner, deal with the same disease. And if love binds them, it's not much exaggeration to say that they both have it.

Parkinson's sufferers in the United States number above half a million, and fifty thousand more are diagnosed each year. Balancing those grim numbers are almost equal ones for care-partners who share the burden of the yoke—half of its weight, and perhaps, toward the end, most of it.

Though a great many women have Parkinson's, I've been speaking with you from my personal experience with it and from what I've observed of the other men in our support group. Every one of us has a primary caregiver. In one case, it is an adult daughter; in all others, it is a wife.

And so, with Anne at my side, I want to talk now about what Parkinson's costs have been beyond me—what it has cost us as a loving married couple; and what it has cost Anne, a strong and independent woman, to be both wife and care-partner. We both believe that this book wouldn't be complete without such a chapter.

There's this about my Anne: early life made her the strong woman that she is. Her childhood was, by any standard, fiercely demanding. By her testimony, Anne's father was cool and emotionally distant; and from the time Anne was six, her poor mother was already showing signs of a progressive mental disease.

"As a little girl, " says Anne, "it was pointless to ask Mother if I could go out to play. There'd be no answer, or a baseless one. I learned to say, 'I'm going out to play,' and then do it."

A brother and sister did her real parenting, each about ten years older. But when they went off to college, Anne was alone to deal with her plight and to make of herself a responsible, strongly motivated adult.

And what a job she did! Fine school grades led to college and a bachelor's degree. Then, because the Masters in studio arts were not then available in her area, she headed south to earn an MA in painting and drawing at the State University of Iowa, and then, at the University of Cincinnati, an MFA in painting with a minor in art history.

Teaching brought her east, first to be Artist-in-Residence at St. John's College, Annapolis; then to stints at the University of Maryland and several other colleges.

Divorce left her alone again when she was almost thirty; but my Anne, bless her, pressed on. Over the next dozen or so years, she continued teaching art but also developed in Annapolis a very successful one-woman graphic-design business. (I've always loved its name: "In Cahoots.")

That's the woman that, two years a widower, I met in the early '90s, just before pulling up stakes in Maryland and moving north to Central New York. We two visited back and forth, grew steadily closer, and married in 1997. You can read all about that in another book, *From Fly Creek* (North Country Books, 2005).

For the first decade of our marriage, Anne and I hiked together, traveled to Europe together, cooked and entertained together. We enjoyed movies, concerts, and the opera; and together we worked our small farm. We told friends that Anne was Flora, and I, Fauna: She tended the 2,000-square-foot vegetable garden, and I wrangled the heifers, sheep, pigs, and poultry that we raised over the years. Geese were the worst, with turkeys a close second. Pigs were the most fun of all.

Of course we were both involved in harvesting, butchering, freezing, canning, pickling, and drying our bounty. And we organized neighbors each October for a sauerkraut party: a hundred pounds of cabbage ending up as gallons and gallons of sauerkraut shared among us.

I needn't have worried about Anne finding her place in our country community. Over our first decade, she was an officer in Rotary, a board member of the farm extension service, president of the Chamber of Commerce board, and a tireless fundraiser for local causes. Anne also entered politics and now is in a second term as a Town Councilperson.

In that first decade, I got immersed in the community, too. I headed the local historical society, helped get National Registry status for Fly Creek, served on the board of Cooperstown's venerable Mohican Club. And I continued as a columnist for the local paper—over eight hundred columns written to date. As a Quaker recorded minister, I did regular counseling at the county detention center and spoke from pulpits around the county.

The book that I mentioned above (my writing and Anne's delicate pencil-drawn illustrations) had us touring the area for readings, signings, and sales of prints of Anne's lovely drawings. It was a busy, happy time.

Of course that bustle of activity changed when Parkinson's moved in with us. Both of us had to retrench from a variety of services, and both of us realized that it was not just I that had Parkinson's. We were yoked as one by our marriage vows and, fundamentally, by our love. We both would bear with Parkinson's.

It remains to tell you about the classic push-and-pull between us that Parkinson's both caused and somehow refereed. And also about the deepened challenge when, three years after my first tremors, Anne was diagnosed with breast cancer. The next chapters are about our dealings with each of these, but I'll tell you now: we've done it all, yoked as one.

Who's in Charge Here?

As of this writing, I'm about three and a half years past diagnosis of Parkinsonism. I also noted earlier that, by the time a diagnosis takes place, the disease has been under way for seven or eight years, with a steady diminution of dopamine production during that whole time. That means, sadly, that I started losing ground to Parkinsonism only three years after Anne and I were married.

From that time and across the seven years before diagnosis, I was undoubtedly showing increasing symptoms of what was to come. But until the hand tremors appeared and led to close testing, there was no reason to suspect Parkinsonism.

Poor Anne! She'd married a vigorous man of fifty-nine, one managing his own household and flocks of farm animals. He cooked meals, sheared sheep, birthed lambs, butchered chickens, built sheds, repaired roofs. He climbed ladders, cleaned out rain gutters, cut and raked hay, hauled it to the barn. He was a great match for Anne since she herself was ready to do all of that and more. What a woman!

Things went downhill in me slowly at first, as dopamine slowed production in the back of my brain. I'm guessing that Anne (not I) began to notice changes after about three more years. I showed signs of forgetfulness, distraction, disorganization, and even clumsiness that weren't part of the earlier Jim.

As years progressed, so did the symptoms. Without my realizing it, my speech softened greatly, to the point that Anne continually had to ask me to repeat things. Of course my reaction was that of many men: the problem can't be with me!

"Sweetheart," I said, "I'm getting worried for you. You really need to get your hearing checked."

She did, and came back with a gleam in her eyes. "Perfect hearing!" she said. "Perfect!" she repeated. "I guess the problem's elsewhere." And of course it was.

After my diagnosis, we both faced a jarring adjustment. "I had been thinking awful things," Anne confessed. "I thought you'd stopped loving me and were trying to drive me away." Now, suddenly, she realized that, however frustrating I'd become, it hadn't been by choice.

My own adjustment was in confronting a downhill slide. Medicines could ease some symptoms, but nothing could stop the decline.

My first reaction was to vow to man it out: to do as much as I could for as long as I could. I would stay an active, self-determining person until such life qualities were beyond my control.

And there begins, friends, the challenge that comes to every couple that faces one partner's diminishing judgment, and perhaps, eventual dementia. (I say "every couple" because Parkinsonism is not the only chronic disease that raises the challenge.) Because Anne and I know the classic push-and-pull so well, we both think it's important that we offer ourselves as an example of it.

The dynamic is surely the same if the patient is a woman, but challenge is especially hard for both parties if the man is ill. We men are, after all, a fragile sex, despite all our strutting and chest pounding. The thought of giving up any degree of self-determination throws us into panic.

"Of course," we insist, "I'm still safe in my driving! Of course I'm still safe in cooking a meal! Of course I'm not going to take a walk and get lost! And I'll certainly recognize the time when I can't safely do such things!"

But (dare I admit?) in the backs of our minds we're

asking, "*But will I?* Will I only give in when I've hit a tree or, God help me, a person? When I burn up a dinner or perhaps the kitchen? When I find myself wandering in our own beautiful woods, befogged, with no sense of where I am or who I am?"

And for the care-partners, those scary questions are not in the *backs* of their minds. They are in the very front. As are more:

"How can I protect my beloved from what's happening to him? How can I support his dignity and still keep him from injury and maybe injuring? Should I jump up at every loud noise from another room? Should I go looking for him if he's slow returning from the garage or the barn?"

So far, so good for Anne and me. She watches and accommodates but tries to do it with tact. And I'm appraising myself constantly. I have already curtailed my driving, and sometimes I decide I shouldn't drive that day at all. I tell Anne where I'm walking or leave a note for her. And I feel self-confident in doing so.

But what happens if judgment suddenly fails me, if prudence suddenly flares and burns out? What's to deter me then?

That's Anne's nightmare, I know. And hence her insistence that I err on the side of prudence, always. And my ersatz-macho response? "Don't mother me!"

Sometimes, in sheer frustration, we find ourselves yelling at one another.

Neither of us can offer a solution to the problem; we can only describe it. What does help is to objectify it as much as possible. If we catch ourselves yelling, we usually sit down at the kitchen table or by the woodstove. We describe, as best we can, how each of us is feeling. We express sympathy for the other's position. And we hug. It's better then. But we know full well it's all going to happen again.

We talk about other things, too. Since neither of us has any children, several years ago we hedged ourselves with long-term health care. The policy allows for home health care as well as nursing home expenses. That's a comfort.

But what changes will have to be made to our home as my physical condition worsens? Ours is a 1794 post-and-beam farmhouse, a truly charming structure that's been fun to restore and fill with period antiques. It is not, however, the house for someone who already bumps into chairs and stumbles on the edge of oriental carpets.

Some furniture has been moved and some carpets rolled up. I'm very sad to see this happen to my home and especially to Anne's. But those are minor changes. What to do about a tight, steep staircase and doorways too narrow for a wheelchair? What about the forty acres, the fence lines, the shrubs and trees I can no longer give proper care?

We love this place, both of us. But what's to become of it and us?

Of course that question isn't unique to us; it reflects the ordinary human lot. But sickness and uncertainty do have a way of sharpening its edge, don't they?

When a Second Shoe Drops

It's almost inevitable. Since Parkinsonism most often strikes people in their sixties or seventies, the odds are very high that a spouse of about the same age will experience a health crisis of some sort, too. It may be a fall, causing a broken arm or hip. It may be a heart attack or a stroke. It may be a tumor or an aneurism. And the fact that the newly afflicted is already the care-partner for a spouse makes no difference. Nature is benignly indifferent to such a fact.

But imagine the blow to my Anne when, in spring of 2010, she was diagnosed with breast cancer.

I've told you briefly about her admirable, even heroic biography. She raised herself beyond a household of emotional coolness—and even mental illness—to make an astoundingly successful woman of herself. Others might have been paralyzed for life with anxiety, dreading that they would always be alone, in danger, without help.

Not my Anne. Any anxiety she countered by firm, positive action. She got an education. She became a recognized artist and teacher, and then a successful graphic designer. If any residual anxiety prowled around the outskirts, she just walled it out with a successful, truly joy-filled life. (Back in Annapolis, she was known to many as "Dancin' Annie;" always ready for sing-alongs, always ready to fox trot, polka, or samba the night away.)

But now, breast cancer. Not a potential challenge from outside, mind you, but a malignancy within her very body. And at a time when her husband was less and less able to offer her support—when she was caring for him.

Oh, my poor dear! If ever there was proof that rain falls on the just and the unjust, here it was. Anne was caught in a deluge that should have driven her to her knees. But it didn't.

A routine mammogram had turned up the cancer, and a team at our regional hospital, Bassett Healthcare, wasted no time in responding. Bassett has a kind of breast-cancer SWAT team, and the very next day she was called back for a sonogram, and four days later for a biopsy. That same day we sat down with a surgeon who gave us a leisured, detailed explanation of what might lie ahead. When the biopsy proved positive, we were back for another careful, extended explanation by the radiation oncologist. We left those sessions shaken, but sure we had a superb team behind us.

And indeed we did. Anne's lumpectomy was on March 22, less than three weeks after the mammogram. The removed cancer was localized, without any lymph-node involvement; her prognosis is excellent. But because of the lump's size, Anne opted to have chemotherapy followed by radiation. The treatments took the whole summer, but reduced the likelihood of recurrence to eight percent.

Through it all, Anne soldiered along, bless her, with the amazing support of the Bassett staff. Nurses, doctors, technicians all treated her with real human concern. They know her name, call her by it, listened to her intently.

When their treatments were finally done, we two went off to a cottage on the coast of Maine for a week. We rested, ate lots of lobster, reveled in scenery almost painfully picturesque. And we came home restored in spirit.

Anne is almost her old self again in joy and energy. Her beautiful hair is already back to a kind of Leslie Caron length; many of her friends say she ought to keep it that way. Anne's husband is relieved, very happy, too. But what was he like through the worst of her times?

Well, he remained the same old bloke he was before her cancer: sick himself, and slipping downhill. But yet he felt stable, serene, still able to support his beloved and sustain himself. Was he ever wrong!

He misled himself, you see, because he'd been through this experience before. His dear first wife had been hit with cancer, and he'd been a trooper through the whole process. True, toward the end the Hospice volunteers cornered him and ordered him to go away for a few days. "You're running on empty," they said. "You're about to fold up, and there's enough sickness here already."

They were right. I reluctantly left Gwen in their good hands, drove from Maryland up to Fly Creek, New York, climbed into bed and slept twenty-four hours. I had been running on empty. And that was Jim twenty years ago and in good health, not Jim at seventy-one and a Parkinsonian.

But I'm a man, after all (i.e., short-sighted and over-confident), and so I continued to pretend that all was well on shipboard. I was at the helm, confident, steering a steady course. What I didn't know was that a mutiny was brewing below decks.

I was so worn down that finally my crew wouldn't take it any more. They blew off the hatches, swarmed the decks, knocked me literally flat on my back. I ended up in Bassett Medical Center several times, once after our Fly Creek First Responders had scooped me up from our living room floor.

On one of these occasions, my every indrawn breath sounded as if I'd swallowed a clarinet—a reedy, ghastly squawk that made me think the end had come. But still I felt calm! I could pray quietly. What *was* going on?

Panic attacks, that's what; brought on by exhaustion, and at the worst possible time.

Anne, already into chemo, insisted on coming on the first trip to the ER. As I lay on a gurney in a cubicle, she sat by my side, bare head covered in a do-rag, her face masked, hands in plastic gloves.

"Anne, love, you shouldn't be here!" And that was true.

Chemo had knocked out her immune system, but here she sat in an ER, in a sea of free-floating bacteria.

"Go home, please," I said. But the chemo had suddenly made her deaf, too. She sat unmoved, unmovable. Bless her.

When I was better and next saw my counselor, I asked him if there was such a thing as a subterranean panic attack. Could one feel calm and still be falling apart? His answer was a smile and, "Sure can!" And then he ticked off four or five anonymous examples from his own clientele.

What those frightening months taught us, and what we want to share, is how suddenly a care-partner can become someone needing care. Ironically, shaky Jim was shifted to care-partner, and he crumpled under the job.

And we learned how such a possibility should be planned for. In fact, we thought we'd planned. As soon as we had Anne's diagnosis, we started trying to foresee upcoming needs. What we didn't see was her Jim knocked to his knees in short order. I won't forget that lesson and offered it recently to another man whose wife has just been diagnosed with metastasized cancer.

He's a quiet, good-humored man with a strong sense of self-possession. When I asked how he was doing, he said, "Don't worry. I've got everything under control." I had to answer him gently.

"Don't kid yourself. I kidded myself, and it made things worse for Anne and me both."

As I've said, neither Anne nor I has children; her family is in western Canada, mine down in Maryland. What sustained us through those awful months was the constant care of friends. My own fellow Quakers set up a round robin of cooking; every week, one of them would deliver a big casserole that would cover several meals.

Other friends from Fly Creek and Cooperstown laid on food, too. And, wonder of wonders, hamlet neighbors not only finished planting Anne's enormous garden but even returned all summer to weed it, too! That sort of generosity left us not just deeply grateful, but humbled by so much human goodness.

If you find yourself in our kind of situation, I hope you are blessed with family close by, or generous friends who will come to your aid. Absent such resources, you may have to hire help. You'll need it.

We're also left aware that a second health emergency could happen again, from some other cause. And whatever time has passed until that should occur, it will surely find this Parkie worse off than now, in need of still more support.

Of course we'll prepare as best as we can. But all the while, I'll be saying, "I lift up mine eyes to the mountains, whence comes our help. Our help is from the Lord, Who made heaven and earth."

And ultimately it is, whether directly or through the hearts and hands of loving family and friends.

In for the Long Haul

You know the truism: You really can't lay claim to your rural home till you've owned it at least a half century. That's how it is in the country—not just around here, but in any rural area. If you've only owned a place for twenty or thirty years, others will still call it by the former owners' name.

I do it myself. If I'm trying to explain where Anne and I live, I can joke and say we're at the dead end of Cemetery Road. But if I want to clinch the matter, I have only to say, "We're in Stanley Stucin's place."

"Oh, sure," people smile and say. "Nice people, Stan and Frances."

I'm sure they were. Frances, we're told, was a warm, energetic woman who raised chickens and a big garden, and pretty much kept up the place herself. Stan evidently lived life at a more measured pace. About my present age when I met him, he was a lonely widower anxious to get out from under "Stone Mill Acres" and carry on with the rest of his years. These, it turned out, were sadly few.

Anyway, if Anne and I manage to hang on here for a few more decades, the eventual new owners will get more than house, deed, and Anne's richly composted garden plot. They'll get the need to explain that they're living in "the old Atwell place." I like that.

Meanwhile, we two are making a move to establish a permanent place in Fly Creek. We're planting our flag, as it were, by buying a plot in the graveyard that's in sight from our driveway. That seems apt, too.

Judy Cook, superintendent of The Fly Creek Valley

Cemetery, is searching the maps for us, looking for a vacant single plot up in the old section, beneath the big evergreens and hemlocks. (We both plan to be cremated, so a single plot will do just fine.)

"I'll turn up a nice one," said Judy, "dry, and without a lot of roots." For no rational reason, I like the idea of "dry," but a root-free plot seems more of an advantage to the hole-digger. Maybe that's what Judy was thinking, too.

I first explored that sprawling old cemetery in 1977, just after my late first wife Gwen and I struck a deal with old Stanley for his house. One autumn morning I was wandering around far back among the graves when, emerging from the mists, there appeared a giant granite stone inscribed "ATWELL." I looked around and saw similar inscriptions. A whole passel of Atwells lay resting there. I went back to the house and told Gwen we'd picked the right place to buy. We were expected.

I asked Judy Cook to look for a plot at least a little distance from those Atwells to avoid confusing any future genealogists. A Maryland Atwell, I'm separated from those local, very distant kin by at least six generations. I found that out with Mabel Atwell, who taught a few of the Cooperstown generations herself, drilling them in the old subject complements and subjunctive clauses. (Mabel, bless her, is now part of that past too.) We researched it together in the census rosters.

It was the redoubtable Mabel who made the definitive judgment. She clapped shut the book of rosters, planted her fist on it, and declared me a shirttail cousin to her late husband. And that was that.

If Judy can swing it, I wouldn't mind a plot near one of Fly Creek's Civil War casualties, since a couple of them actually died in my native state. A tall obelisk standing just above the winter vault records a young man killed at Sharpsburg. Another has a Fly Creeker dying only four miles from my own home. In an exchange of ill prisoners, he'd been brought by steamboat up the Chesapeake to recover his health at Annapolis before being shipped north to home. But he worsened and died.

In my boyhood, that huge cornfield outside Annapolis was still called "Camp Parole."

The most moving Civil War markers, though, are on the graves of two brothers, killed in battle within a year of each other. Side by side, the stones can bring tears almost a century and a half later, for their inscriptions must have been chosen by a desolate father. On the earlier stone, a carved hand extends down, holding the handle of a hook. From the hook dangles a single link, for a second link has broken free from the first and is falling away.

On the later stone, the second link has also broken free; the hook hangs empty. The second link has fallen to the earth. It lies rejoined to the first.

I hope our old house stands for another two hundred years. I hope eight or nine more human generations shelter under its sturdy roof. Lots more, I hope, will feel pride of ownership, though, like us, they'll really only have a short-term lease. But meanwhile, Anne and I have made plans to stay in Fly Creek, just up the road, under those handsome fir trees.

This hamlet is home and always will be.

High Drama by Bowen's Toe

I'm just back from Lake George and a week's sharing with hundreds of Quakers from across New York State, and from parts of Connecticut and New Jersey, too. It's always a relaxing time, full of shared quiet as you'd might expect, but also full of leisured rocking-chair conversation on a broad veranda, singing there in the evening, and laughter at kids that leap and gambol across the broad lawns like herds of elands on the veldt.

There are business meetings, too, long and sometimes tedious. But by and large the week is one of relaxation with old friends that one sees only once a year.

An optional activity that I truly love occurs each morning at seven, down on the boathouse's covered porch. About twenty early risers gather there for a half hour of sitting with silent attention to the calm spread of Lake George, the range of hills beyond the far shore, and, above their rolling green, a steady armada of fleecy white clouds, usually sailing south to north.

I never miss those sessions of quiet. They contrast so peacefully with the splashing of more Spartan Quakers who are not far away, taking early morning dips in the frigid water. That's not for me. I want the blessed quiet, the view, and the swallows cutting graceful arcs in front of us, sometimes flying under the porch's roof, right over our heads.

The second morning, however, I saw a life-and-death struggle, right there on the boathouse porch. I was sitting in a line of wooden rockers, and Bowen Alpern, the Quaker to my left, had a large bare foot resting on the second rail of the rustic balustrade. He was lost in his own quietness and hadn't seen the small spider web just above his big toe, tucked in the angle of top rail and upright.

In the web was a proportionately small spider, itself tucked well into the corner, waiting. And soon a midge flew right into the web and stuck.

If you've read this column over the years, you know I'm prone to pathetic fallacy—to projecting human feelings into animal and, on really zany days, into trees and shrubs as well. And so whatever other thoughts were nourishing my spirit were lost as I watched the ensuing struggle.

At the first tug, the little spider was alert. I imagined some kind of spider adrenalin exploding through it, making it lead into action with an unspoken "OK!" It started down the web, full of spider excitement. "OK! OK!" But then, "Oh crap!" The midge had broken free, tearing out a section of the web.

The spider was very still for a few moments, but then it began an attempt at repair—a half-hearted one, I thought. (Had spider disappointment given way to spider depression?) After too few circles of spinning around and across the ragged hole, it headed back to its corner. But it had hardly arrived when another midge (certainly not the same one!) struck the web and stuck.

"OK!" I imagined in a tiny, tinny spider voice. "OK! OK!" And then, again, "Oh crap!" For the second midge had torn free, leaving still more damage to the web. What happened then really worried me. For the spider started for its corner without the first attempt at repair. Oh, my. What was now needed? Therapy, medication? But no such things exist in the bug world …

Whatever the need was, it solved itself in a way that shocked me. A dragonfly sailed straight in from over the lake, struck the web, and carried off the whole thing, little spider included. The insect rose on sparkling wings and flew between Bowen's and my heads. After it was gone, I stared.

There were lakes, hills, processing clouds unchanged. There was Bowen's foot and big toe, unmoved. But the miniature drama, stage, and actors were gone, as if they had never existed.

I sat back in my rocker. What to make of that? I could think solemnly on "Nature, red in tooth and claw." I could consider that best-laid plans of spiders and humans "gang aft agley." Or I could search the event for what 14th-century mystics called "correspondences," parallels between earthly events and the vast world beyond our senses, or perhaps messages from that world. How did that one-act drama speak to me?

I opted for the last, weighing what the spider's life and plight might have to say about mine. This meant starting with some discrimination.

I don't mean mindless, repellent discrimination like that based on skin color or religion. I mean careful analysis, the very basis of rational conclusions: comparing and contrasting items as to their similarities and their differences.

Well, what about me and that spider? Of course there is the huge difference in size. I'm maybe four thousand times larger (more, after the Silver Bay's excellent desserts). But measure us both against the scale of the Earth, and that size difference becomes insignificant. Measure the Earth against the Universe, and it's that difference that's become too absurdly vast to have meaning. The spider and me? Forget about it!

And there's little to note in differences between the substance and motivations of T. S. (tiny spider) and me. We both have live bodies and grow, fix parts that are injured, reproduce and nourish ourselves. We both have locomotion, though T. S. easily had me beat with all those legs. And we had the twin motivations of pleasure and pain.

The standout difference, I guess, is humans' evolved capacity to reason. That means that we don't live in an eternal "now," as did T. S., but can trouble ourselves about the past and about the future. It means that we can syllogize our way from "all living things die," to "therefore I will die." No spider loses sleep over that.

But, hey, quite apart from my projecting onto the tiny spider, we two have lived the same life. (Sorry to suggest that T. S. is in the past tense, but if that dragonfly, disentangling itself, spotted the spider, there's no doubt of the outcome.) I have spread a lot of webs in my day, then crouched in the corner, hoping to snag power, money, happiness. And lots of times my web has been torn and I've felt too despondent to make repairs.

And a day will come with the dragonfly that rips loose my final web and carries me off with it. I hope that at that moment I won't be saying, "Oh crap!" I hope to say, "OK. OK."

"Don't look at him, Marlene!"

First, glad tidings: Our Blue, who has long had his mismatched eyes fixed on gaining the grand official status of a Therapy Dog, has made it! He's now certified as a polite and useful visitor to hospitals, nursing homes, schools, and other places where an affable dog's visit would be a value. I know you send your congratulations to Blue—and to Anne, who led him through the training, and especially through the last few lessons. These involved reacting calmly to wheelchairs and walkers, and to sudden loud noises and unexpected hugs from burbly women. (I don't think Anne was subjected to the hugs.)

Though Anne should receive a "Dog-Owner Hero" patch for her efforts, the goodies all go to Blue. With the recognition, he'll get a certificate suitable for framing (to be hung under the kitchen table, his favorite hang-out) and a dashing scarf that has "THERAPY DOG" imprinted on it. The scarf worries me a bit, since it brings to mind Isadora Duncan.

You remember Isadora's sad end in 1927. A bohemian modern dancer given to melodramatic gesture, Isadora was climbing into a low-slung Bugatti convertible with her lover *du jour* when she tossed the end of a very long scarf toward those seeing them off and trilled, "Goodbye! I am off to glory!"

The scarf tangled in the back wire hubcap of the car; as it roared off, Isadora's neck was instantly broken. A warning is here, I'm sure, for us all, though I'm not clear on what it it might be. "Watch out for European sports cars," perhaps?

Or, "Affected gestures may endanger your health?" Anyway, I'm keeping Blue out of pricey convertibles and making sure he has no loose ends to tangle into anything, including wheelchair wheels.

As befits a dignified Therapy Dog, Blue is very affable toward his new roomie, Simon the cat. They're not exactly pals, but Blue is uncomplaining when Simon drinks from his water bowl, and Simon sits at a polite distance while Blue crunches his kibble. They do touch noses when passing, a civil gesture that some human grouches might well emulate.

We've kept Simon inside these first few weeks, and he's been quite happy exploring the house and stretching himself out to impossible lengths as he luxuriates in front of the woodstove.

He is a gifted sleeper, as are most cats. They aim for eighteen hours of shut-eye in twenty-four; and Owen of blessed memory, especially in his last years, topped that number routinely. Simon hasn't reached the goal but shows great promise. Every night he pads up the stairs to sleep with me, and during the day he climbs the same wooden hill to join me in my naps.

Some Parkinson's patients, including me, sleep an outrageous amount, largely from exhaustion from the disease's other symptoms. It's not unusual for me to sleep a twelve-hour night, and then add to those two more during the day.

Quick arithmetic will show that my conscious life is frequently reduced to ten hours out of twenty-four, into which I must fit three meals and various kinds of therapy, plus hug my wife and pat our dog and cat, plow snow, and tend the chickens. And, of course, write to you regularly. I love doing the last-mentioned, but I'll admit it's a slower process than it once was.

During my hours of sleep I have Simon's enthusiastic company; Anne says we not only have a certified Therapy Dog, but a Therapy Cat, as well. I would agree. There is something wonderfully soothing about his purr as he settles across my knees if I'm facing up, or onto the small of my back.

He's very forgiving, too. If I roll over in the night and send him bouncing onto the floor, he'll sit by the window awhile, collecting himself, and then jump lightly back on the bed and back on top of me.

During the daytime naps, we leave the shade up on the south-facing window as a nod toward passive solar heating. And so I must settle down wearing a long-ago gift from British Air. From back in the halcyon days, when even coach fliers were given little kits to make them more comfy, Anne and I each have a fine complimentary sleep mask to block out light. (From those kits, we also have several miniature toothbrushes, really too small for human use. I'd gladly give them away if we knew some gnomes.)

My sleep mask is a sober black, but Anne was given one that might match a special-occasions negligee. It's crimson satin with black rubber bands, and both eye-covers are slightly convex; I think it looks like a bra that Barbie Doll might order from Victoria's Secret. So it's creepy to pull that one down over my eyes. But, then, I can't see it in the sudden dark, and nobody else is around but an uncritical Simon.

I have to wear the satin Barbie bra during siestas with the cat because the sober black mask is kept in the glove compartment of the Prius. This is for my use when Anne and I go to a shopping center and I opt to snooze while she gets what we need. Indeed, if I lean back my seat and put on that black mask, I'm zoned out in seconds.

I'd never think of wearing that vulgar Barbie rig for car-sleeping. I can just imagine reactions of passing people. Here comes, for instance, a tired mother, dragging along behind her a spirited six-year-old. The little girl spots me in the car and asks, "Mommy, what's that old man wearing on his face?" The mother, stops, stares, glares. "Mommy, what is it? It looks like ..."

Mommy has her by the arm now. "Don't look at him, Marlene! That's just what he wants!" She drags Marlene past my open window, pausing only to hiss in at me, "Dis-GUST-ing!!" There's enough breeze and venom in that mid-syllable for me to feel both.

Nope, no Barbie bra in the car for me. If it comes to that, I'll just have to wrap my face in a scarf—something like Isadora's.

Give the Man a Medal

After awarding recognitions to every other member of our place's domestic staff, it's time to give one to myself. All these awards, of course, (so far, to Anne, Blue the dog, and Owen the cat), are to boost morale and team spirit amongst us. And, for the same reason, here comes my award.

But wait, you may say. How could a man of such natural modesty present an award to himself? It would run counter to his entire life of admirable virtue. Of course I have an answer. One of my virtues is a profound humility, and it's humility that requires me to present the recognition of my feat.

According to Aquinas, a medieval specialist in, among many other things, the categories of human virtues and vices, *"Humilitas veritas est,"* i.e., "Humility is truth." Being humble is not a matter of denying one's strengths and playing up one's weaknesses, as did Dickens' repellent Uriah Heep; it's judging oneself objectively and noting both the one and the other.

And so, because, unlike Uriah, I am truly "a very 'umble person," I must recognize my recent achievement and also give it public recognition. Please join in applauding my recent accomplishment in senior acrobatics. But let me first provide some background.

One of Parkinsonism's more diverting symptoms is very vivid dreams and even hallucinations. In the last category, for instance, I once lay wide awake on my bed in the middle of the afternoon and glanced down to see Brian Bean, who installed our solar panels, standing at the foot, grinning at

me. When I sat up and said, "Hey, Brian, what are you doing here?" he vanished.

Another time (again mid-afternoon) I started to get off
my bed and faced my speech therapist standing nearby. He
was dressed, not in his white Bassett lab coat, but in a
Union army uniform, complete with jaunty campaign cap.
Again, he vanished when spoken to.

On both occasions, I stress, I was wide awake—as I was
when I glanced up at the ceiling to see a pink hairbrush
drifting along just below it, gliding effortlessly like a pink
fish seen from sea bottom. We have no pink hairbrushes in
the house, I thought to myself, and I addressed it.

"You're going to disappear, aren't you?" And it did,
forthwith.

The dreams are just as vivid. They are long and involved, and I remember their details by the wheelbarrowful.
Lately they've been based in tedious searches, often against
impossible deadlines. I'm in Kennedy Airport, for instance,
finally at the front of an endless line at the airline counter,
checking my bags for a London flight. "Your passport,
please," says a bored young clerk, and in panic I realize I've
left it back home in Fly Creek, safely on top of my bureau.
Or, wait! Did I absentmindedly chuck it into the suitcase
with other stuff on the bureau?

"Stop that suitcase!" I shout, since my bag is already
tagged and trundling away on a conveyor belt. The riled
clerk does, hoists it over to me, and orders me out of the
way. I crouch between the snaking lines, and open the case
to display the chaos inside. (I'm not a good packer.) I
burrow among papers, books, socks, jockey shorts, shirts,
shoes, medicine vials. I dig frantically for that blue passport.

People in the line snicker. A kid says, "Mommy, why's
that man throwing around clothes in the airport?"
Everybody laughs. I wake up.

But the dream that should win me a medal took place
outdoors. I'm standing in a gravel pit where I used to shoot

skeet as a teenager. I'm dressed in suit and tie, staring in horror at my watch. An important Washington figure is speaking on my college's campus, and I'm to introduce her in fifteen minutes. The campus is about four miles to the west. I set off at a run, tie flapping over my shoulder.

I stumble and scuff my carefully polished shoes. I fall twice, ripping the knee right out of my suit pants. But suddenly I'm running along the shoreline of Spa Creek, near my home. I've run ten miles in the wrong direction! Desperate, I wheel around and run north, run and run.

Gasping and tattered, I come up against an eight-foot chain-link fence. Beyond it, about a mile away, I can see the college's buildings. "I've got to scale this thing," I blurt, and start to do just that. As I drag myself to the top, I see that the only way is to throw one leg over and the rest of me after it. I do so.

As I fall, I whack my head on something, there's a thunderous crash, and I'm lying on my back on the bedroom floor. I have thrown myself out of bed. I'm wrapped in half of the bedclothes, dragged along with me. And I'm wearing my sleep apnea mask, its long plastic hose curling up and away from my face like the trunk of an elephant about to trumpet.

"I'm on the floor," I think groggily. "I threw myself over that fence and landed on my bedroom floor." No college in sight now; no distinguished guest leaving the campus in a huff. Things were coming clear. "I'm in Fly Creek, damn it, on my back on the floor, a hose sticking out of my face. I'm an elephant in blue pajamas, half wrapped in a red blanket."

By now Anne (who understandably sleeps in another room) is at my side. "Are you hurt?" she says.

"No, no," I say with forced good humor. "Somehow I rolled out of bed," I say, chuckling.

Rolled, hell! I threw myself out, right leg first, and over an eight-foot fence. But no need to add all that.

Anyway, I deserve a senior acrobatics award for that performance, and I'm giving me one. Why, if that had been in formal senior competition, I'd have won at least a bronze medal. (Whacking my head on the bedside table, you see, would have cost me some points.)

Healing Hands

Some Parkinson's folk get real relief from some of their symptoms through acupuncture. I haven't tried that myself but want to comment on its value to introduce another alternate healing technique. It's one that has benefited me greatly.

Our tiny hamlet of Fly Creek, New York, is blessed by the presence of an excellent acupuncturist. I visited with him in his comfortable office near our old trolley station. Justin Deichman is a quiet, centered man with evident deep knowledge of alternate healing techniques. I'll say at once that Justin, like me, doesn't see "alternate" as meaning replacement for western medicine. Rather, he sees the varying techniques as possibly valuable adjuncts to what western medical science can do for us.

Justin explained that the acupuncture he practices is most well known for its high development among the Chinese; in fact, it is practiced in folk medicine around the world. Through measureless years of experiment, various cultures have discovered that specific points on the body, when stimulated by light placement of needles, can provide relief to a variety of human ailments—physical, emotional, psychological, spiritual.

The explanations for why this should be vary from culture to culture. The most common metaphor is that of bodily "ports" which, when functioning properly, admit the energy around us. That energy field ties us to the rest of creation and nourishes us just as do more obvious energy sources like good food, clean air, and sunshine. (Sunshine is the most obvious external radiant to us of health and energy.) The stimulation of the tiny acupuncture needles revitalizes the sluggish ports and makes them more efficient recipients of energies.

Of course many will dismiss acupuncture and the like as just New-Age shamanism and clients of it as simply trapped by gullibility. But here's a point to consider.

Western medical science of a hundred years ago now seems incredibly naive to us; and surely in a hundred years the medical science of our own time will seem just as naive, just as shortsighted. In light of these simple facts, if other cultures, through millennia of experience, have discovered healing techniques that work, why dismiss them simply because we don't know how they work and can't yet name or measure them? That doesn't strike me as a scientific approach. It strikes me as childish arrogance.

This same judgment applies to reiki, or healing energy work. Again the underlying premise is that we live and move inside a sea of energy fields. Some, like the sun's light and warmth, are perceivable by our senses. Others, like the waves of electronic communication, constantly surround us though we can't grasp them immediately with our senses. And here's the basis of a very useful analogy:

For us to grasp and make use of energy fields beyond our sense's ordinary powers, two things are essential. The first is a *transmitter* that changes to something we can perceive, and then channels the energy to—what? To attuned *receivers*. That's us, oh best beloved!

No real practitioner of healing energy work claims to be more than a sensitive transmitter. Yep, there are charlatans out there, ones who claim that they are not mere channels but possessors of super energy themselves. If I weren't a card-carrying Quaker, I'd say pox on all such fakes who undercut and debase a real source of healing! I'd be tempted to lay hands on them myself!

Sorry about that sudden un-Quakerly outburst, but the

true practitioner of this art readily admits that what talent she or he has is not based in self, but comes from outside and above. It's a gift, just as is a musician's perfect pitch or an artist's special sensitivity to color, texture, and shape. And the ability meets all the tests of a gift: It's valuable. It's freely given to its possessor. And it's undeserved.

A deeply gifted energy healer named John Calvi says the receiver and user of the gift is just a conduit, nothing more. He'd better think of himself in the most ordinary of conduits: a cardboard tube from a paper-towel roll or, better, an empty toilet-paper roll that energy speaks through.

Pretty mundane image, isn't it? But John's point is this: Unless the practitioner accepts and holds to that humble role, he'll just get in the way of the transmission.

Just as important as the practitioner's recognition of his humble role, however, is the client's openness and acceptance of a role as receiver. Almost a thousand years ago, long before the world became aware of transmitters and receivers, St. Thomas Aquinas said, "Everything that is received is received after the manner of the receiver."

What that awesome monk meant was this: Unless we are open to reception, it won't take place. And how it takes place will be qualified by what we are as receivers. And what kind of receivers we are, is the sum total of our life's experiences to date. Good stuff!

So: if we are open to the possibility of energy being channeled to us, and if we are positively receptive to it, then we may very well benefit by it.

But another caveat: beware of the charlatan who claims that he or she not only possesses powers, but that those powers can absolutely cure.

Nonsense, I say. Every integral practitioner of reiki or related fields that I've known has readily acknowledged that their work can produce a temporary effect (easing of symptoms, etc.), but that the effect will wear off.

Well, I say, so what? I'm reminded of evangelist Billy

Sunday's response when a reporter said that salvation for some of his followers didn't seem to last very long. "Neither does a bath," said Billy, "but we take 'em anyway!"

My bottom line: Don't hesitate to explore this interesting possible help. Find somebody good and give healing energy a chance to help you.

Learning the Ages of Man

My gosh, it turned out to be true! Recently I've talked to ace reporter Casey Campbell, who turns columnist himself each week on this page. Casey confirmed the shocking truth: he has never been in a *bona fide* barbershop. Every haircut this twenty-something has had has been the work of a unisex stylist.

Well, it's all right, Casey. You've turned out just fine anyway. And besides, I'm guessing your whole generation of young males has come of age, somehow, without benefit of the barbershop experience. You've all made do without the peculiar bonding, the identity building that used to come from a specific source. I mean a monthly visit (at least) to one of those scruffy shops, most of them lit by humming, sometimes flickering neon tubes.

What else can I tell you about those shops? Well, in summertime, certainly during my Annapolis boyhood, barbershops could be hellishly hot. No air conditioning back then (you had to go to the movies to enjoy that). Instead, a barbershop would have a huge pedestal fan, six feet high, standing alone in a corner, or maybe several oscillating fans mounted high up on the walls. The fans churned the heavy air, rattled magazine pages, made tufts of cut hair roll like tumbleweed across the worn tiles. The heat was largely unaffected.

But the fans did plague the barbershop flies. These had been drawn to the entry by the cloying smell of pomades and unguents; and with each single patron, a half-dozen flies buzzed in. ("Screen door's there to keep 'em from escaping," old timers would say.)

The blasts from the big fans would throw the tiny flies wildly off course as they sailed around the shop, and some old gents spent their waiting time on the alert, batting them out of the air with folded newspapers. On Saturdays, fly stats were kept and money made on bets.

Six decades later, I can still see one old geezer sitting forward in his chair, eyes bright and head thrust forward like a turkey's, his folded newspaper at the ready. Someone would call out, "Here comes one, Bud!" and the entire room would watch as the old man tensed like a terrier, then swung.

"Aw, bad luck, Bud. That bugger veered when he saw your arm move. But, by damn, he's got a story to tell his grandchildren!" And the old boy would grin and realign his false teeth, gone askew from his swing. Then he'd gather himself and wait for the next low flier.

But most of the flies, after bouncing along against the tin ceiling, ended up gathered inside the front window, battering heads against the sun-bright plate glass. The broad window seat was littered with dried corpses and the bodies of addled, dying flies. The latter lay on their backs, trying to take flight but spinning instead among the deceased.

Enthroned in the barber chair, swathed in a striped sheet, I had all that to watch, plus, if I were lucky, a shave in an adjoining chair.

For a shave, the customer was dropped back almost prone, feet raised. In preparation, the barber swathed the customer's face with a hot towel right out of the chrome steamer. While the moist heat softened the beard, the barber would hone his razor on his chair's leather strop. Then he'd work up a thick lather in a crockery mug.

I loved the slip-slap of the stropping, the clickety-click of the shaving brush handle against the mug, the rhythmic scritch of that straight razor as it cut through hairs. I can still hear them all in imagination. And I can also recall the shout of pain and annoyance if the barber nicked something other than hair.

Once, after a third nick, a client roared, reared up, and jumped from the chair next to me. He wiped the lather from his face with his striped sheet, ripped it off and threw it down at the barber's feet. Then he made a uniquely Italian gesture at barber Calabrese and, pressing his wounded earlobe, stamped outside through the entering flies.

The glowering Calabrese, chin jutting like Mussolini's, dismissed the man with a contemptuous, "Sicilian!" Being from Calabria, the Calabreses viewed Sicily as a mere misshapen rock. To them, the Italian boot was poised to kick it the length of the Mediterranean. Along the wall, the waiting customers murmured over the incident. But in the next barber chair, I kept very quiet. Great-grandpa Onofrio Geraci, after all, had fled his native Sicily just ahead of Garibaldi's conscription officers.

But what great stuff for a kid to witness—competitive fly-swatting, Italian drama, and all from the middle of the action! Plus a haircut. Plus a smelly pomade scrubbed into my scalp that was guaranteed to make me irresistible (well, sooner or later.)

I just hope today gives kids something similar to feed their imaginations, their identities; something that will plant memories for a lifetime. For instance, I don't know who that fly-swatting old geezer was; he may be a composite formed by my memory. But as I approach his age, I love the old boy for his spirit, his zest. He played his part in the barbershop's helping me get an early grasp of something. In college I learned Shakespeare's name for it. In *As You Like It*, after "All the world's a stage," he outlines the very barbershop drama in which I played a part.

Shakespeare calls it "The Ages of Man."

Dear Old Earth, Still Turning

We experienced a fine adventure during our first week in England, but I'd like to tell you about one in the second week first. (Did that make sense?)

During the first week we were visiting the Throwers, down in Chichester near Portsmouth. At week's end they kindly drove us up to Buckinghamshire and turned us over to Paul and Beryl Witheridge, genealogical buddies of Anne. Like the Throwers, Paul and Beryl showed us a great time: she, a superb cook, laying out splendid meals (including a salmon en croûte I'm going to try reproducing very soon); and he, an Oxford graduate, touring us around the university and the old city.

Because Paul knew that Anne and I were both fans of the TV series, "Inspector Morse," he created a "Morse" pilgrimage for us, leading us around to area pubs and seating us right where Chief Inspector Morse had sat, berating his patient subordinate Lewis. And Paul and Beryl also conspired to remedy a problem from an earlier visit by Anne and me, maybe ten years ago.

Back then, I'd been driving her through Salisbury Plain, spouting pedantry about historic spots we were passing. Ground mist steadily thickened into fog just as we approached a major attraction: the Great White Horse of Uffington. I was excited about artist Anne seeing this awesome figure, carved through the turf and into the limestone face of a great hill over three thousand years ago. The figure is stylized and seems timeless; it almost portends those spare paper cutouts made by Matisse during his last years.

And here's what astounds me: The local folk have carefully maintained the Great Horse, even as religions and attitudes have changed around it, for thirty centuries. The country folk have always regarded it as sacred, and neither medieval church nor the 17th-century Roundhead icon-oclasts dared to move in and destroy it. Hurray, I say, for a sense of the sacred!

The horse, all sharp angles and vital energy, is a football field in length from nose to tail. Seen from below against the lush green of the mountainside, it's breathtaking. That's what I wanted my Anne to see, even as the fog thickened. We crept along the road below it.

"There it is!" I shouted, keeping eyes riveted on the obscured road. "The Great White Horse, right up there on the hillside!" Anne's response was laconic. "What hillside?" she said. And what hillside indeed? There was no hill to be seen, much less a prehistoric horse.

When I told the Witheridges about that disappointment, they privately decided to remedy it. Without Anne's know-ledge, we three took her on a leisured drive to the Great Horse, approaching the site from the far side of the round-ed mount on which it is carved. We parked halfway up the steep slope and then trekked on by foot.

I can't tell you my personal elation to find that, though at some cost, I could still climb a height as I had for so many years of hiking in England. And when we reached the mount's broad top, I felt, as Brits say, "over the moon!" The windswept top was several acres of stubby grass, and grazing idly across it were dozens of sheep. As I walked through them, they gazed up with eyes wondrously innocent of intelligence or guile.

I said "Hello, sheep!" repeatedly, and I got a few baa's in response.

When I walked toward the far edge of the hilltop, still another wonder opened before me: the whole of Salisbury Plain, or at least a 180-degree panorama of it. A thousand feet below us, it spread out for hundreds of square miles, blanketed by farm fields. There were crisscross roads, quaint church spires, and clustered village houses. Rising smoke suggested cozy hearthsides indoors.

What an experience! Even if it should be my last time on such a height, no matter. It will live on within me. I'll imagine that climb and the wind-blown hilltop, the grazing sheep and, oh, most especially, that breath-stopping view of the dear old Earth, still steadily turning.

My Anne, meanwhile, had been walked to another spot of the mound's edge and realized that she was standing just above the head of the Great White Horse. (Later we walked down beside it, steadily more amazed by its size and artistry.) Anne was delighted, as were our hosts.

Nearby stood a much younger couple; she was turning slowly, eyes closed, arms extended. When I glanced toward her partner, he explained. An old myth claims a wish made and backed up by that ritual at the Horse's head would surely be granted.

I considered, and then, set aside closing my eyes and spinning. I'd have stumbled and bounced, tail over teacup, down a thousand feet to the plain. But then I turned to see my Anne, bless her, making her own slow spin.

I didn't ask what my love's wish was. Didn't have to.

Here's Your Easter Basket

As Easter approaches, some bleak news on the candy front. Cadbury's, the staid old British firm that produces those splendid cream eggs, has itself been gobbled up by the American giant, Kraft. The Cadbury's name will remain on the cream eggs; but in the future, be careful. Some may be stuffed with Velveeta.

In face of the takeover, and as a comfort to you and to me, I'm offering you your Easter basket a week early. Its contents are two final stories from our recent England trip. The events occurred within minutes of one another; but there's some other, more elemental link between them that I sense but just can't pinpoint. Maybe you can.

Our first English week was in Chichester, that dear old cathedral town not too far from Portsmouth. Early one morning, I rode the bus into the town center, intending a quiet day of enjoying a place that, again, I never expected to see again. On arrival, I opened my own day of celebration at a small restaurant down a narrow, cobbled side street.

Wickedly, I ordered a classic British "cooked breakfast," a lovely spread of comfort foods and, I suspect, a real maelstrom of cholesterol. Not something you'd want very often, it features a couple of fried eggs, British bacon, baked beans, a grilled tomato, and, if it's the real thing, a link of black pudding. The last is hog's blood, simmered till it darkens and thickens. It's then made into a link sausage. I'd call it an acquired taste, like the Scots' haggis or the Norwegians' lutefisk. No black pudding for me that day; I have *some* self-control.

The first of my two events occurred as I walked toward the 11th-century Chichester Cathedral, ambling along a slate sidewalk between the cathedral and West Street. To my left and down a slight slope, a sweeping spread of lush grass stretched to the building's side wall. To my right, alongside the street, a bus shelter held a queue of patient, waiting Brits. An overcast day, and comfortably brisk. So much for setting the scene. Now the action.

From the bus shelter, a lad of about four escaped his mother and galloped down the slope onto the greensward. It was cold enough that Mum had him sealed up in a hooded snowsuit. Well, as you know I'm a sucker for kids; I stopped to watch his progress.

The lad picked up a fallen twig about the length of his arm, and was at once deep into some man-against-monster fantasy. He brandished the stick above his head and, considering his very small lungs and voice box, produced a creditable battle cry. "ARRRGH!" he roared and charged an invisible, much larger foe. To my delight he vanquished it, ending with a foot clamped on its chest and a flourish of the stick. Then he turned toward further adventures—and spotted an ancient and half-sunken tombstone, rising out of the grass only to about half his height.

Again came his "ARRRGH!" as he charged this new monster, one dragging itself out of the earth. "Uh, oh," I thought. "He's going to try to leap that stone." I saw at once that the snowsuit legs were too baggy to allow it, but leap he did. He was partly successful.

The lad pivoted over the small stone and ended hung up on it, head on the ground, legs waving behind. No roar now; just a little boy's panicked cry. He struggled and freed himself to fall sideways onto the grass. I thought sure he was going to cry. But even as his face puckered, he saw some old man watching him from the sidewalk.

This warrior wanted no sympathy. He picked himself up, found his stick, and brandished it at me. "ARRRGH!"

he roared, and galloped off to attack the cathedral wall. Oh, thanks, lad! What a show!

Then, in minutes, the second event. I walked on and rounded the base of the bell tower. Between it and the cathedral main entry was a statue I don't remember seeing before. On a tall granite plinth and made of burnished steel, it represented Saint Richard of Chichester, a 12th-century bishop of that very cathedral.

A holy and compassionate man, Richard took special care of the poor. He was much loved, and was canonized not long after he died. His tomb in the cathedral was a pilgrimage site for hundreds of years—until Henry VIII decided that he needed to break the resistance of wealthy Catholics down there in Sussex. He commanded them to dismantle the tomb and turn over to him its precious and bejeweled gold decorations.

That didn't stop the pilgrims, of course. But after one of Henry's later successors was beheaded by the Puritans in 1649, Oliver Cromwell decreed that this papist practice must, like all others, be quashed for good. And so a godly crew arrived at the cathedral and spent a long day demolishing the stonework and desecrating the shrine, all to God's greater glory.

When the Puritan wrath faded from the scene, a new Saint Richard's shrine was built and is reverently tended by the cathedral's Anglican clerics, members of Henry VIII's fairly new church. *O, mores! O, vita!*

A short prayer that the saintly bishop Richard composed nine centuries before was carved into the statue's big stone base. As I stood reading it, I realized I was memorizing the prayer. It was entering my heart.

The prayer's first short paragraph was thanks for all of one's life's blessings and for Christ's bearing pain and insult for humankind's sake. Then the prayer eased away from formality, addressing Christ directly as savior, then friend, then, movingly, as brother. And there followed lines that seemed to leapfrog forward to the 1970's, then back to Saint Richard's time:

"Let me see you more clearly, love you more dearly, follow you more nearly, day by day."

Yes. The writers of the New Age "Godspell" had high-jacked Richard's prayer, though I'm sure the saint didn't mind. (And, of course, no copyrighting back then.) But if you're about my age, you'll remember those gentle words and the lilting melody that accompanied it:

"Day by day, day by day, these three things, O Lord, we pray." Then, in those three phrases above, a summary of our whole Christian pilgrimage.

Now, how do those two events outside the cathedral—that little boy warrior, so vulnerable but so full of zest; and the twelfth-century bishop and his eloquent prayer—why are they bonded in my spirit?

Beats me, friends. And so I'll just leave them in your Easter basket. Let me know if you figure them out. Meanwhile, Easter blessings on you, day by day!

A Vacant Place Against the Sky

The metaphor is an old one. Someone dies whose strength and integrity seemed to tower over the rest of us; a person whose goodness has given shelter and comfort to hundreds of others. Then death comes and we are left diminished, bereft. We feel as if a great tree, part of the scenery of our lives, has toppled and left a gap on the horizon.

That was the feeling of many around here, and indeed around the whole state, at the death of George Badgley of Fly Creek.

A Quaker's Quaker, George was blessedly free of dogmatism, deeply reverent in following Jesus' teachings, tolerant and forgiving of others, and good-humored in the face of all humans' frailty, including his own. All this, and physically a towering oak of a man, broad-shouldered, with a handsome face of such strength that, even in great old age, it seemed hewn from granite.

The first time I sat with him after his series of strokes had begun, I tried to suggest to him how much I'd learned from his example over the years. He smiled and thanked me, and said it was hard to hear that. For George, an impulsive giver to others, found it hard to grasp how much his gifts meant to his beneficiaries. Humility was that deeply engrained in him.

That day on his front porch, I didn't want my words to sound like a summing up, a goodbye. But, as George's body steadily weakened, I wanted that still-keen mind to know my gratitude. So I told him about visiting a grave in Wales, resting place of a man who'd towered in County Merioneth as George had in our midst.

Dafyd Lewis was a cousin of my late wife's, and his son Gwilym had taken us to visit dad's grave. The handsome slate gravestone was inscribed in Welsh, and so I asked Gwilym to read and then translate it for us. Gwilym read with the eloquence born in all the Welsh; that rich, impenetrable language rolled out of him like falling water. Then he translated the epitaph of his beloved father:

"Night has fallen on Dafyd Lewis. But he plowed his furrow straight, and now he has followed it back home."

George Badgley listened to that epitaph and nodded slowly. Then, speech slurred, he deflected the implied compliment from himself by reaching for a plowing story from his boyhood. Debbie his wife sat by us. She surely could have recited this story by heart; but, lovely woman, she waited to the end of each labored sentence before restating it, all the while looking at George to confirm her accuracy.

Between them, they told us how George, even as a farm boy, loved poetry. He memorized and recited many great works, and he even tried to compose his own. While he plowed a furrow, he was also composing; and he would often stop at the end of a furrow to align a couple of newly shaped lines in his mind. Once, he said, laughing, the lines were something like, "Do not shirk/ your day's work ..." But, that long-ago day, his reverie over them had been broken by his father.

"George!" he called out from across the field. "You're resting that horse a bit too much between furrows!" And, chastened, young George went back to his plowing.

Even in the Best of Families

Here's another sheep adventure for you, friends. Again, it occurred back when we were keeping a small flock year 'round. If you choose to draw a moral, do so; but if you just enjoy the story, I'll be well satisfied. For drama's sake, I'll keep the tenses as they were when I first wrote the story.

At last count, four black lambs were bouncing around in our sheep shed. They vault over one another's backs, dash out into the snow and back again, then drop onto their elbows to pound away at their mothers' udders.

I say "at last count," because Sophie, our third ewe, remains enormously pregnant. She is bulging like a barrel about to burst. Sophie, who is likely carrying triplets, looks as broad as she is long; and she is dragging around an udder that is, well, Dolly Parton-esque.

I go out to the shed three times a day, hoping each time to find more lambs. No luck. There stands Sophie, other mothers' lambs bouncing around her, her head down and miserable. I wish I could do more than say, "Poor baby!"

Long-time readers of this column might be muttering, "Wait! He shouldn't be getting lambs in February. Don't they usually come in late April or May?"

Yes, that's true, friends. And that would be the case if the pregnancies had followed on the visit of David the rent-a-ram, who was with us back in November. His visit should have meant lambs in five months, sometime in late April. But, as it turns out, David's work had already been done for him, back in August.

Did I hear a gasp? Did I just hear someone whisper,

"But who …?" OK, here's the plain truth. Last year's lambs had among them a couple of little rams. And before they went off to summer camp at the end of August, those rams managed to get a next generation going. Yep. Shades of Oedipus Rex.

And, yes, a better shepherd would have prevented that. Within the appropriate number of days after those ramlets' births, he would have applied the elastrator, which puts an elastic band around their begetting equipment. Somehow this shepherd missed the time for doing that. And so he went through the summer, hoping for the best. But the best was not to be.

Those rams, randy as teenagers by last August, followed nature's lead; and here I am, tending lambs in sub-zero cold. And waiting for Sophie to worsen the problem—in an overnight snowstorm, probably, with gale-driven drifts blocking the sheep shed door.

But if our flock is the cause of local embarrassment, not so of another four-legger at our place. I mean Blue. He continues to advance in agility training and now can weave among poles, rush through tunnels, and clear obstacles with the best of them. His next class, I think, will have him tap dancing and performing simple card tricks.

But last week revealed still another talent in this triple-threat dog. He's a *bona fide* therapist, and not just because he's licensed as such. The dog is a true healer.

Anne and I have a good friend living at a nearby nursing home; he's Blue's good friend, too. In past days, Joe Ranker, a grand old-timer known to hundreds around here, would never drive by our place without watching for Blue. If he spotted him, Joe would pull into the yard and hand him a dog biscuit out the van window. Blue, of course, soon knew the look and sound of that van, and he'd plant himself by the roadside, waiting for Joe.

A stroke put Joe in Otsego Manor some months ago; and, although he is doing quite well under the excellent care there, I know he misses Fly Creek and especially his philanthropy to its dogs. And so my Anne, bless her, decided that she and Blue should both visit Joe. She phoned ahead and got clearance, then headed for the Manor with the leashed dog at her side.

And here's the wonder: Though he'd never been to that nursing home before, he at once recognized it as like the hospital. When he trotted into the lobby, the energetic Blue stopped, sniffed the new environment, and at once quieted himself. At Anne's side, he padded softly down the long hallways.

When they got to his room, Joe was asleep in his wheelchair, his hand draped limply over its arm. The dog knew his friend at once. He padded over and put a wet, cold nose into Joe's palm. Joe awoke with a start, looked, then smiled radiantly.

"Blue!" he said, and the dog nearly threw himself off balance, wagging his tail. He sat down next to the wheelchair as Joe scratched his ears. Then, while Anne and Joe visited, Blue flattened himself on the floor, sighed, and fell asleep.

"As we left," said Anne, "we swung in and out of several day rooms. Lots of residents patted him and admired his soft coat and mismatched eyes." And each time the dog, sensing the frailty of his admirers, played his role to gentle perfection.

"Bring him back again!" said the staff at the front desk. And we surely will.

So forgive us, please, our misbegotten lambs. (It happens, as they say, in the best of families.) Pay heed instead to Blue. By raising smiles and good memories, he confirmed an old truth: "Dogs are instruments of grace." To which I say, Amen.

Speaking from Deep Inside

Last year Anne took a pilgrimage north into her past. No, not to Canada, but to Gloversville, New York. I was pleased to go along since the past was in small part mine, too.

Back as academic dean at Anne Arundel Community College, I'd start each semester by signing a stack of about five hundred contracts for the part-time instructors who taught a third of our courses. I had no idea that, each time, I was confirming the contract of the woman who has since so blessed and renewed my life. Anne's was just another document for me to sign.

In that same stack each semester was a contract for Anne's good friend and colleague Peg Swartout. At that point I knew Peg no more than I knew Anne. In both cases, the Humanities chair had done the recruiting and interviewing, and his judgment was excellent. It took fate to bring Anne and me together (read the book!), and through Anne I met Peg.

Anne always described Peg as an artist's artist. Indeed she was. Her skills and enthusiasms burst the limits of her training as a painter and foraged through the whole world of crafts. Indeed, Peg made no distinction between fine art and craft. She just saw the world, rejoiced in it, and spoke the joy in whatever medium seemed best to embody it.

But she wasn't a dabbler, this Peg. She'd topped her Master of Fine Arts from the Maryland Institute with work at three prestigious craft schools. The end product was a disciplined artist and craftswoman completely at home with oil and acrylics, but who was just as at ease with potter's clay, weaver's yarns, papier-mâché, and, indeed, with often making the paper on which she drew. And her buoyant enthusiasm made her a great teacher, too. Small wonder she and Anne were buddies at Anne Arundel!

And not just at the college. While both taught and pursued their own art, Anne also branched into computer design and publishing. While Anne managed "In Cahoots," her well-known design business, Peg was producing materials for over forty exhibitions in the Mid-Atlantic area— some with Anne as a fellow exhibitor.

Their deepening friendship continued across a quarter century, and they kept in touch even after Anne moved north to Fly Creek. And here's kind coincidence at work: Peg grew up in Gloversville and often visited there with her husband Ron.

We last saw them in 2004, when Peg's sister Pat brought them to visit us in Fly Creek. Two years before that, they had been in a terrible car accident that left Ron permanently injured. Peg recuperated, but in the middle of lively supper conversation at our house, she let drop that she wasn't driving anymore. Then she added brightly,

"They say I have Alzheimer's, but you don't think so, do you, Ronnie?"

That gentle man said, "I think you're doing fine, Peg."

And she was doing fine, still rejoicing in her art, still exhibiting. But in fact Alzheimer's was closing in on her, and she was well aware of its progress and implications.

What took us to Gloversville last week was a lifetime exhibit of Peg's work. She has now slipped quietly beyond any ability to express her artistry, or even to recognize her past work as her own. Her sister Pat told us of Peg's daughter sitting with her, guiding her fingers across the textures and shapes of her carvings, her weaving, her graceful clay pots. Perhaps Peg, smiling gently, didn't know what they were; but she loved the feel of them. And, who knows? Maybe they spoke back some of the love she had put into them.

Peg couldn't be at the lifetime exhibition organized by her sisters. The pieces were on display in what had been a grand bank at Gloversville's old Four Corners. Now the Chamber of Commerce lets out the vast marbled lobby for special gatherings, and the high walls and light from the windows above them make it perfect gallery space.

The works that Pat and her sisters had chosen, scores of them, were displayed along the sweep of the marble walls and on tables and stands throughout the lobby. Anne called me over to one table that held a thick binder. It was Peg's clipping book of the forty exhibitions, and my Anne flipped some pages and stood smiling.

"Recognize her?" she said. There, standing with Peg and a third exhibitor, was my Anne in her late twenties. I was already happily married back then, but that girl would have caught any man's eye.

With Anne, I followed the sweep of Peg's work around the high walls. Anne remembered every one, and at one point noted that a few were out of actual chronology. But, no matter. The sheer energy and joy radiating from those works possessed us both, right up until the last three or four. These dated from after Peg's supper with us at our house and showed a brave woman coming to terms with failing cognition.

The first a collage she had titled, "On the Bridge," was almost painfully evocative. Peg had merged together small reproductions of most of the world's famous paintings of individuals on bridges, including Edvard Munch's "The Scream." She put in place that image, that figure with hands pressed against temples, to frame a face without hair, eyebrows, or any individuating features. What was Peg seeing as she did so?

The next painting was of a serene woman draped in bright yellow. From the top of her head exit blossoms, buds, leaves, all spreading and thinning into a blue sky. It is titled, "Where Am I Going?"

The second-last painting is not representational and it might seem inchoate at first glance. It is not. One color explodes into another as it sweeps across it; and shapes are at once dissonant and perfectly apt.

The last painting is of a seated woman, motionless, staring neither into past or future. I believe it is a self-portrait.

I hope that textures, colors, shapes still drift within a silent Peg, crossing, mixing, creating kaleidoscope images. I hope they sometimes fall into shapes that make her spirit gasp in delight.

Oh, the beauty!

All Lines Down, but Still There

Years back I may have told you the story at the end of this chapter in a column; but, even if that's so, I need to retell it. It follows strongly on last week's column. And further, as Quakers say, the story "speaks to my condition."

Last time I talked about Anne and I going to a lifetime-achievement exhibit of works by her colleague and friend, Peg Swartout. Peg is deep into Alzheimer's now, past even knowing her own artistic accomplishments. So her two sisters, bless them, arranged a major exhibit to honor their sister's joyful love of life and her embodying that love in art.

Peg will never know of the exhibit and what it has meant to those viewing it, especially my Anne, who knew many of the paintings and art objects and had watched as some were created. No way now to thank Peg for that beauty she produced. She's alive still, but almost all lines of communication are down. She responds to a loving touch with a gentle smile, but otherwise she lives deep, deep inside herself, her radiant mind now a flame turned very low, barely flickering.

And, oh, friends, that statement "speaks to my condition." As you know, Parkinsonism is diminishing my action in the world, and may eventually close down my awareness of it.

I have the classic symptoms of Parkinson's disease, but extra symptoms suggest that the final diagnosis will likely fall elsewhere in the Parkinsonian family. That's a highly dysfunctional family, and progressive dementia comes with many of the member-diseases. And so, in Peg Swartout's present state, I am possibly seeing my future.

Do I think about that a lot? You bet. But thought and prayer have brought me to terms with it. If such is to be, it is meant to be. The way I end will come to me from God's hands, just as did my coming to be at all.

If I have dread, it's not of dwelling in silent blackness, as does Peg. I dread the half light just this side of the darkness, a time of confusion, of loss of words and memory, a time when I may not know my dear Anne's name. A time of wandering from room to room, sure that something must be done, struggling to recall just what it is. A time of living in gray fog but still knowing that my most personal human needs are now tended to by others. I do recoil from all that. But I accept it in words as old as Christianity: Thy will be done.

But about that story. I'll almost call it a miracle, so comforting has it been across my last twenty years. It was a message I needed back then and need again now.

Back then, my first wife was dying. Gwen put up a fierce fight against what ended up as pancreatic cancer; so strong was her will to live that the disease was eighteen months in killing her.

It began with a misdiagnosis, but an understandable one. Gwen became jaundiced. Our doctor, a close friend, ordered a sonogram; sure enough, her gall bladder was full of stones. We were referred to a surgeon, the kind of cool clinician that can give that specialty a bad name. The surgeon removed the gall bladder and, as a standard final step, ran a small rod down through the common bile duct to dislodge any stones that might be there.

Tragically, as that rod slid the length of the duct to its opening into the duodenum, it broke through and spread a cancer partly blocking the opening. No one's fault, really. A cancer there is as rare in women of forty-seven as is breast cancer in men of that age.

Back home, Gwen seemed to improve steadily. Then, after weeks, the jaundice came back. When I phoned the cool clinician to tell him, he said flatly, "That's impossible. I cured her."

Just as flatly, I answered. "The whites of her eyes are lemon-colored." I didn't add, "you arrogant fool!"

An endoscopy confirmed that the cancer by then had metastasized, ascending the bile duct to attack the pancreas, and also settling, it turned out, in her liver and brain. There followed a long and drastic surgery that left Gwen unable to digest anything without first downing a half-dozen pancreatic enzyme tablets.

"No need for chemo," that same surgeon said at that point. "I've removed the cancer."

In not many months the cancer had spread into Gwen's liver and her brain. In her last months she was lost to me. Morphine sulfate held back the agony, but, along with the brain metastasis, it made her a wordless ghost, motionless on the bed. I was sure that I'd never hear her rich voice, her laugh again.

But, here's the miracle: I did.

In the early hours of one morning, I was lying awake next to Gwen, who was still as a tomb effigy in her drugged sleep. Then, suddenly, in a warm, conversational tone, she began to speak. I froze, daring not to move a muscle.

From somewhere deep within her, Gwen had taken an imagined telephone call, probably from some former New York colleague at Albany or Alfred. From her responses, I'm presuming the colleague was asking about her living in Maryland and about her new college.

"Annapolis and the Chesapeake are great!" she said—with all the warmth and spirit I thought were gone forever. Whatever the colleague said next brought a hearty laugh from Gwen, who answered, "No, no, the equipment is great! And I really like the students here."

The next question brought the impish, ironic tone that

was Gwen's hallmark. I'm guessing it was, "How are the new bosses?" For Gwen's reply was to pause, and then ask, "You got about an hour?"

Then, that beautiful, bell-like laugh again. Then, nothing more. Silence.

I lay on my back, tears coursing down and into my ears, stunned by the gift. Cancer had ravaged her brain, knocking out all lines of contact. But somehow my Gwen was still inside, intact.

As perhaps Peg still is. As perhaps I will be.

Woof, Woof, Woof-Woof!

It had already been a busy morning. I'd headed outside with Blue and a plastic bag, resigned to following behind him and collecting a specimen for the vet. (Dogs have physicals, too.) But we'd hardly cleared the screen door when things got exciting.

Blue spotted four deer beyond the fence in our east field and, too good to be true, a flock of wild turkeys in the south field. He streaked away from me, woofing mightily, and ran the length of the east field's fence. That sent the panicked deer streaking south and right into the turkeys, which took off in their own clattering flurry to land in trees outside the field. The deer raced on in arcing leaps down the field, cleared the fence, and disappeared into the woods.

What a show! And Blue enjoyed it too, especially as I shouted "Good dog!" repeatedly. He pranced a bit, paused, turned thrice in a small circle, squatted, and provided the perfect denouement. All that running must have done it, I guess. I couldn't have asked for more. I mean, anything else.

When he was done, Blue did his usual pawing, followed by rocketing around the field in a victory lap, his ears and tongue flapping. He ended at my side, panting, with an expression that clearly said, "What a good dog am I!"

As he certainly is. Witness his steadily more disciplined approach toward the sheep, whom he loves. I've told you how he used to enter the sheep's paddock with me, merge into the flock's midst, and accompany them to their food trough. But now, on his own, he's realized that, at that moment, he can't pretend he's a sheep; he's a working dog.

He enters the paddock with me and then stands by my side as the baaing sheep, anticipating breakfast, come thundering in from wherever they were grazing. An old git shouldn't block the way of six sheep at eighty pounds each, and so I stand to the side and wave them toward their inner yard and the trough, shouting, "In!" Most go, though a couple of dimwits always want to follow me to the feed barrel instead of going to the trough. (Canny old coot, I keep clear of those milling bodies by standing by the barrel and throwing the feed over the fence and into the trough, picking just the moment when all the bodies and heads are out of the way.)

But even after hundreds of feedings, as I say, a couple of dimwits still try to follow me to the barrel. And here's where the new, improved Blue moves into action. He trots around behind the miscreants and deftly woofs them to and through the gateway to the inner paddock. And there, wondrous to say, he stops and stands, with no attempt to follow them and pretend he's a sheep at the trough. What a dog!

After Blue and I returned to the house, I carrying his gift for the vet at full arm's length, I turned to the breakfast dishes while Blue settled himself under the kitchen table. Anne, upstairs dressing for a meeting, had left the "Today" show on in the living room, and the principals were yammering cheerily about upcoming guests.

One of the guests must have been a baseball star, for as they chattered, an engineer cut in with the opening bars of "Who Let the Dogs Out?" That's an irresistible song, and so, scrubbing egg yolk enamel off a plate, I sang the repeat of the title line.

"WHO LET THE DOGS OUT?" I bellowed lustily— and nearly dropped the plate when, from under the table, my line was followed by "Woof, woof, woof-woof!" And right on the beat, mind you!

What to make of a dog that can do that?

Blue has a few weeks off from his usual therapy-dog

visits to Bassett Hospital patients because of the run-up to the general election. No, it's not Blue that's running this time; it's Anne, running for the town board. But his celebrity might make him an apt candidate in the future. After all, he can melt hearts with his soulful eyes, especially because of the black streaks under them that look so much like mascara smudged by tears.

It's almost embarrassing to see Blue capitalizing on his looks when we go to the Fly Creek General Store for coffee. I tie him at the geezer bench outside, and he climbs on the bench to watch my every move through the big plate glass window. My traditional seat is just beyond that glass, and there he sits, studying my every move, especially if I raise something to my mouth.

As I return his gaze, I see many incomers pause to scratch his head, and I see their mouths move as they say, "Hello, Blue!" Then they come in and bawl me out for leaving that lovely, sad dog outside and alone. If I don't watch carefully, some soft touch will buy a sausage muffin and sneak it out to him.

But I can't fault him for his behavior with the public. In many ways, his performance on the geezer bench parallels what he does at Bassett Hospital. There he pads up to a wheelchair, puts his head on someone's knee, and gazes up with those soulful eyes. Patients laugh with delight, and they sometimes even cry, perhaps as Blue evokes memories of dogs long past.

Good for him, I say! And, in his lingo, "Woof, woof, woof-woof!"

It's a Matter of Time

As to my shifting a weekly column to one that leapfrogs to every second week, I owe you some explanation. What is driving the change, friends, is narrowing time limits, and on several fronts.

I'll be writing to you half as often because it's become twice as hard. Not in garnering materials, certainly; life in Fly Creek still blesses me with armloads of it. But these days I sometimes freeze at the keyboard. It's not that my hands won't work, but that my mind seizes up. Then I just have to sit back in my chair and wait for my brain to reboot itself.

But other Parkinson's symptoms are gaining on me, too. More trouble with stumbling and with short-term memory. Tremors and shakes abound, both day and night. The docs explain that all the jouncing around is like lots of tiring aerobics, and hence my voracious need for sleep. I'll typically sleep a twelve-hour night, and then lose a few more hours to sleep during the day. At least once or twice I've matched Simon the cat's gold standard of eighteen hours sleep out of twenty-four.

That much sleep doesn't allow for a lot of consciousness during the day; maybe ten hours, on the average. Inside that time I must manage to say my prayers, hug my wife, pat my dog and cat, feed and water the animals, read the mail, keep up with the news, visit with friends. Oh, and write the column.

Those shakes and quakes coming at night, by the way, are a further sign that I'm now wandering in a notoriously bad place: "Parkinson's Plus," a neighborhood full of thugs that will mug or snuff you on a whim. Multiple System Atrophy prowls there, and so does mad-cow disease, and Lewey body disease, and lots more.

All these bullies carry a grim note that classic Parkinson's Disease does not. Though PD can drain all quality from your life, it won't kill you. These PD+ guys will, and, on the average, within about eight years beyond diagnosis.

And here comes the arithmetic problem: "If Jim is now about three years out from his diagnosis of Parkinsonism, and if, as the end approaches, he must allow for at least two years of severe mental and physical limitation, how many productive years does Jim have left?"

Don't know about your answer, friends, but it looks to me like three or four. To hedge his bets, Jim had better pull off his major goals in that time. He had better be quoting Andrew Marvell: "But at my back I always hear/ Time's winged chariot hurrying near."

Well, I have a couple of big projects in mind, both of them books. And so I'm getting ready to clear the decks, rev the engines, (add other apt metaphors, if you like), and aim all my energies toward getting them done.

The subtitle of one book is "A Book for the Unchurched," and that's exactly what it will be. For there are thousands (millions?) in this country who want to take seriously their spiritual pilgrimage, but who have abandoned formal religion. They have given up on creeds and (to them) empty preaching, but desperately miss the strength of shared worship, of praying and singing together.

And there are millions still in the pews and some in pulpits whose personal prayer has moved them beyond concepts that seem to fall far short of the God they have come to experience. These people have stayed inside the church structures, perhaps because they can't bear to leave them, or perhaps, in the case of those in the pulpit, because they won't walk away from the good they can still do inside the structures.

Nothing of this book-to-be will challenge the faith of firm and committed believers; indeed I hope they might find useful things in it. But they aren't my audience. I want to talk to the expatriates who are feeling their way along an unlighted path in sadness and a sense of guilt, always fearful of a misstep. I want to talk with them about God, Christ, church, prayer, and shared belief. I will speak as a Quaker, but more importantly as a Christian.

I'll tell you more about the other book some other time, if I'm given time enough. But here's a tease: It will be called, "Christ Laughed."

And what if some part of me grinds to a stop before both books or either one is done? Well, so be it. I'll accept that as readily as I have the drive to get started on them. As a Quaker, I see that drive as a leading: an urge by the Spirit that a particular job is one's to do. This one's mine, and I've got to get cracking.

All Spill, All Feel Dumped On

You've long since figured out that the Fly Creek General Store is my second home. I love the dog-eared ambiance and especially Tom Bouton's banter with staff and with the regulars—Gordy, Pete, Mary Ann, Mike, Karen, and a half dozen more who love to laugh and to thrust and parry with one another. What a place! No wonder it feels like home.

At least, almost always. I don't know his name, but there's a guy who sometimes blusters through the door inside a toxic cloud that can smother the fun. I'm guessing his belligerence (head down, shoulders rolled forward, hands often in tight fists) bespeaks a powder keg of anger and frustration inside him. And his talk matches his appearance. He scowls, then growls and gripes about most anything that comes to mind. His team has just lost to a bunch of jerks. He hates his work. Taxes are crushing him. Salesmen try to swindle him. And on and on.

Tom Bouton, bless him, understands this guy; he kids him along, but always with a special gentleness. Tom, I suspect, knows a lot more about him than the rest of us do. We just drink our coffee and wait for the storm to move on, out through the door.

But recently this anonymous man did something so contemptible that I felt like taking my cane to him. I had along my ash cane, bought years ago in England's Lake District. I'd chosen it from a display of ruler-straight canes for two reasons. First, it had a slight double curve in its length. I'd been the last kid picked in a lot of games sixty years ago; I didn't want that cane to end up alone in the display. Second, the cane had a graceful, beautifully grained bole as its grip.

That bole, swung in a long arc, was just what that bozo was asking for. And I'd have let him have it except for my being old and wobbly and easily pounded right into the floor. And of course I'm a Quaker and shouldn't even think of breaking somebody's nose with a cane. So I suppressed temptation at once. But I'll tell you what raised it.

On that morning the man came in and let the door close in the face of a pretty woman who'd followed him from the car. As he headed for the coffee, he called over his shoulder, "You get the Danish and pay."

She did this dutifully as he began to fill the largest of the paper cups, a 24-ouncer. But when putting on the lid, he flipped the cup and dumped a pint and a half of coffee across the counter and onto the floor.

The surly man's reaction, I suppose, was predictable. He stepped up to the deli counter to yell at staff.

"Could we get some towels out here?" he shouted. "There's spilled coffee on the floor."

The tone was what first made me want to grab the cane. Veiled accusation toward the staff. And then the passive voice, exonerating himself. "There's spilled coffee" indeed! But it got worse. He then barked at his wife by name. She was still at the register, halfway down the store.

"Get over here and help with this mess!" She came at once. His idea of help turned out to be stepping back while she dried the counter and then knelt to sop up the floor. Meanwhile, he filled himself another giant cup and capped it successfully.

"There's more under the coffee machine!" he said and then went out the door to their car. When the woman was done, she drew her own coffee and followed him there.

Oh, shame on Quaker me! As that cretin was filling his second giant cup, I was imagining swinging the cane's heavy bole, not at him, but smack down on the cup, squashing it explosively and perhaps scalding him, just slightly. I didn't, and probably not for noble reasons. But that poor woman! What a life she must lead.

And that poor man, too. What a torture it must be to be what he is, and so to miss out on life's joys—and especially on appreciating the love and loyalty of that good woman. If he happens to read this, here's my hope for you, friend:

I hope that you're freed of whatever in you causes you to rage at life. I hope you realize that we're ALL rained on by fate; probably we're meant to get humble from it. I also hope that you catch on that making mistakes comes with our flawed nature as humans. We ALL spill coffee (just ask Tom Bouton); and, again, our clumsiness ought to put us in our place.

Oh, and I dearly hope you come to see that life's greatest blessing is love shared with a dear and loyal partner. You have that, buddy. Be grateful, and tell her so.

I'm also tempted to send a message for your patient lady: if he pulls that kind of stunt at home, you don't need a stout cane. A cast-iron skillet will do the job.

But I won't send that second message. Good Quakers never say such things.

Just Pick the Right Caterpillar

I always forget to mark it on the calendar, and so I'm recording the date right here: On August 5 of this year, the Town of Otsego guys started to build Mount Grit. Their Mack trucks make deep, chesty growls as they rumble westward up Allison Road, straining under the tons of grit they're hauling from the gravel bank.

I love their parade each year, right under my study window. I sit at my desk, comforted that the guys are going to watch out for us again this winter. For as each truck driver slows at our corner and then grinds on up Cemetery Road, he's heading for the growing Mount Grit next to the town garage. I'll watch that hill heighten across succeeding weeks. And before its peak is first dusted with snow, our guys will be ready.

They'll have the big blades on the Macks by then. And with the first ice or significant snowfall, they'll be out there plowing, scraping, spreading, working to keep us safe. Good going, guys! We don't say it enough, but we're grateful.

But why worry about when the crew begins to build the mountain? Superstition, that's why. This time of year I begin looking for omens of the winter it's going to be. I know, I know! It's months before the first snow flies. But now is when the omens begin to appear. You don't have to believe me. Ask any geezer around here.

And as an omen, the date that town trucks start their elephant parade past my house, plus the height of Mount Grit when they're done is probably as good as any. Certainly as good as how early the crickets begin to sing, or how frantic the squirrels seem, or just when the crabapples start to drop.

Gordy Robinson, one of the Fly Creek General Store senior sages, often supplies me with omens, and so does his buddy Pete Costello. Gordy is grand company, full of local lore and strong opinions, and always ready to express both. Pete plays straight man to Gordy; he is poker-faced and quiet. But when he cuts into Gordy's entertaining, it's usually with a real zinger. Bless 'em both! They're worth the price of Tom Bouton's coffee, which is plenty good itself.

When I raised the subject of omens last week with those two, I was almost overwhelmed. Both men opened figurative trunks and started pulling out the omens, piling them on the table. "Rain by seven, clear by eleven!" said Gordy, with a pope's infallibility. And he's right—at least on the days I've remembered to notice.

"When snow backs off from around the tree trunks, winter's done," added Pete solemnly. And, yes, I'll buy that one readily. (I thought better of adding an omen that I read years ago in "New York" magazine: "Rain by noon, dark by midnight." It never fails.)

We three agreed that the trouble with omens is not finding them, but interpreting them right. The town trucks, for instance. Why am I presuming something significant about how early the truck runs begin, or how tall the grit pile gets? Do I think that Shawn and the boys gather deep inside the town garage, faces painted blue, to stir a seething pot of road kill and auger the future? Of course not! Which brings me to a point.

Omens have only the meaning that you give them. The best example of that around here is caterpillars—not the scrawny ones that wreck your linden's leaves, but the fat, fuzzy ones that start clomping around right now, pretending to predict the winter. This week I faced one of those bozos on my back step.

It was striped across the back in black and white, but

that immediately recalled a theological dispute among local seers. Does the black represent heavy snow, or does it stand for snowlessness? Does the white predict blizzards, or does it mean an open winter? Go figure.

And factor in this, too: Is there a significance in the positioning of the black or white, whether it's toward the head or toward the tail? (Caterpillars really don't have tails; they just sort of run out of segments and little feet.)

And what about the ones that are black (or white) both fore AND aft, with the opposite shade, dead amidships? That was the very sort of bug rumbling across my back stoop the other day—heading, mind you, for our back door! Did that mean it carried a special prediction for Anne and me? Are we fated for a personal ten-ton snowflake to squash us flat?

With a shiver, I poked the caterpillar with a fingertip, jounced it 180 degrees and away from us. It stood still a moment while, I guess, its GPS recalculated. Then the insect veered right, described a tight arc, and aimed toward door again. It trundled straight ahead, as a poet said, with "majestic instancy."

Yikes! What to do? Stomping was an option, but people get zapped for killing bearers of bad news. For a panicked moment, I thought of trying to unscrew his head and install it at his other end. But that would only have made for a dead messenger—and a gondola car of bad karma for me. So I picked him up and carried him in my closed hand down to the creek. (He crawled around inside. Creepy.)

There I launched him onto the current on a big piece of bark. With luck, he's well down the Susquehanna by now, heading for the Chesapeake. But I wonder, will he find his way back? Will I yet hear a tiny knock at the back door?

And the caterpillar business gets worse. Gordy says sometimes they come in ALL black or ALL white. What the heck does that mean? Skip the snow tires? Or hoard toilet paper and trail mix? Beats me. Just comfort yourself by thinking that an omen carries only the meaning you give it. That's for sure. Probably. Maybe.

OK, OK. Forget that! The best thing to do is decide what you want. Then watch for a caterpillar that matches it.

Fresh News From the Front

Correction: A while back, I was telling you about the amount of CO_2 not released into the atmosphere last year because of our three solar panels. That figure should have been 4.5 tons. My handwriting's grown so crabbed that I misread my own notes.

That crabbed writing prompts me to another report on life with Parkinsonism. It's a genteel struggle; it pushes firmly, and I push firmly back. No victor so far, though I'm afraid I've lost ground in recent bouts.

Remember, I'm not listing symptoms so you'll say, "Poor baby!" (though that's always welcome). And if you want generalities about the disease, there is plenty of information around. What I can tell you, especially readers who've borne with me for years, is how the stuff feels from inside. That's "the rest of the story."

Now, I know this is thin ice, but I've noticed something about women in casual conversation: They don't mind cutting into someone's sentences or talking right across other women already speaking. None takes offense. Women's social talk (it seems!) sometimes is only excited, reassuring sound that bonds the group.

(Be careful, Jim! Some are clenching their fists!) Of course women engage in serious thought and serious talk. But, when just socializing together, women parallel us guys' joking, "bustin' chops," and punching each other's shoulders. It's all bonding, friends, and just fine. No fault, no penalty.

But with Parkinson's, I can't abide overlapping talk. A

horrendous example for me is the TV show, "The View." It drives me bats. Two women panelists try to raise the tone, but mostly the whole group shouts statements over one another—three and four at once. If a male is a guest on the show, the tone changes; panelists listen to him and to one another, rarely interrupting. But if the guest's a woman, they yank her right into the maelstrom of happy gabble.

OK, I'm backing off from that subject; I feel imperiled. (Remember, I'm old, sick, and maybe not of sound mind.) But here's an example of how the mayhem hits me: Anne and I are sitting on the sofa, reading through the *Oneonta Daily Star*; she got to the crossword first, I have the opinion page.

On the TV, "The View" women are at it. The clamoring gnaws at my attention as my shaky brain tries to hold on to reading; but five outside voices are demanding attention, all at once. And just then my life's love, in all innocence, speaks from the couch's other end.

"Jim, what's the four-letter name of an Arizona Indian tribe?"

BZZZAP! There's no smoky smell of synapses short-circuiting or burning out. It's more like a seizing up; maybe a brain freeze, though not the kind that comes from swallowing too much crushed ice too quickly. But it does hurt, and it benumbs my thought. Sometimes I have to get up and leave, not even answering Anne with, "Hopi, I think." Because I can't think. Not just then.

That's too long a description of a growing symptom. But it is important, at least from here on the inside with Parkinson's.

And more than TV shows do it. I get lost sometimes in ordinary, animated conversation in a social group. I'll be following somebody's anecdote, but halfway through, someone else cuts in with a related story—and someone else sidetracks with a third. My wobbly consciousness still tries to hold onto that first anecdote, and the second as well, and then, BZZZAP!

And here's another symptom to lay on you, friends, one you may see in me even in one-to-one conversation. My face sometimes gets a bit twisted these days, with right eyebrow notably lower than the left and mouth slightly pulled askew. I'm not sneering at you. I just sometimes look that way, and likely it will get worse.

And more: My face is given to random spasms, lips compressing repeatedly, left eye closing in a startling, piratical squint. What's coming may be a classic Parkinson's symptom: facial freezing, where ability to express emotion through one's face is gone. You've seen recent films of Muhammad Ali. PD has turned his charmingly antic face into a frozen mask, just as it has hushed his loud voice to a slurring rasp.

I'm not there yet, and may never be. But Parkinsonism is showing up in my features, especially if I've overdone things. And so, if you note such oddities, don't be concerned. And don't pretend not to notice them. Sharing your awareness makes the changes easier for both of us.

Now, another symptom, odd and somehow endearing. It concerns my toes, antiques now, but a good set. I have never had reason to grouse about them.

But some months ago I awoke to a rustling at the bottom of the bed. "Mice?" I thought drowsily. "Mice under the covers?"

Nope. It was toes. Mine. On both feet they were doing some kind of line dance, waggling sometimes in unison, sometimes in multiple solos. I found I could stop their mischief, as a teacher would an unruly class. But as soon as I turned away my attention, they were back at it again. And they've continued to act in this way, almost constantly, day and night.

It's just another example of lost neural control, but it is distracting and tiring. But as I said, somehow endearing too.

I sit on the edge of the bed in the morning, looking down at those homely feet that I've had for so many years. And there are those toes, line-dancing away, indifferent to me and my will, way up at the other end of me. I have to fight past those wacko dancers to get my socks on.

Sometimes I'll suddenly notice they've stopped; even toes get tired, I guess. I'll try not to rouse them, but how to tiptoe around toes? Then, they're at it again, like baby chicks just awake and ready for action.

So: what I have on my hands (feet) is a set of toes with life and motion of their own. They wriggle away merrily like a game of "This Little Piggy," but it doesn't end with some little pig running all the way home. All the pigs stay right there. They dance and dance.

Heinz Kuhne, Going in Style

"Nothing so reveals a man," someone said, "as the manner of his dying." That's surely ponderous, but true. If one's end doesn't strike all of a sudden, and if one's mind isn't clouded by sickness, a person's dying will echo how a life's been lived.

These recent weeks, I've watched a remarkable piece of dying. It was the work of a treasured friend, Heinz Kuhne.

Heinz had helped his beloved Franzi raise their three kids, all of them now grown up and very successful. He'd run a giant construction business and prospered by it. In later years, he had worked tirelessly with the Boy Scouts, and, more recently, for Habitat for Humanity, using his carpentry skills to help house the homeless. Heinz had lived for sixty-four years with strength, verve, generosity, and a wicked wit. And now he was leaving his life with all those banners still flying.

Heinz had entered Bassett Medical Center Hospital for the last time just a couple of weeks ago. He was fighting pancreatic cancer, and the end seemed near. But Heinz, a take-charge man all his life, was still running the show. Surrounded by his family, he presided over his hospital room; indeed, he held court there. And, blessedly free of intense pain and quick-witted as ever, he waited for death.

Friends came by the dozens, fought back their tears, said goodbye. And they laughed, too, often uproariously. For Heinz was Heinz still, joking them past their sadness.

"I'd better die soon!" he'd say. "This is getting embarrassing! Hey, grown men come in, cry over me, and then

I don't die? I'll have to go hide in Florida, maybe get in the Witness Protection Program!"

But still, Death was the one visitor who didn't show up. And so Heinz and his family kept on celebrating his living. For Franzi and offspring Glen, Chris, and Kathi laid out a buffet in the hospital room, fed each and every one who came in. They hauled in the slide projector and, grouped around Heinz, filled the wall with bright images of their shared life. And filled the room with still more laughter.

Days before death finally arrived, the kids did a glorious thing. They rented an ambulance and loaded Heinz in it. With a convoy of cars following, the ambulance drove north to the edge of the Adirondacks. They pulled up in front of the chalet-style cabin Heinz had only just finished building for them.

The plan was to give Heinz a last look through the ambulance doors. But the medics had caught the family's spirit. They picked up Heinz and carried him into the cabin. The neighbors had seen the convoy pull in and started arriving on snowmobiles. And in the house he'd built for his family, Heinz had a last party.

That night, back at Bassett, he sank into a drowsy half-sleep. And in a few days, Death finally showed up.

I'll remember Heinz from three days before the Adirondack party. He is lying in bed, facing a big poster that his daughter Kathi had taped to the wall. It's a photo of Heinz fifteen years before, a joke photo he'd had Franzi take of him.

In the four-foot-tall poster photo, Heinz is standing in the woods, wearing only blue bikini briefs, posed like Superman ready to take flight. Tan, strong, with hair and beard still black, he's holding his arms outstretched from his sides and clutching a beach towel by its corners. A stiff breeze is billowing out the towel behind him. Heinz is trying to hold a righteous, super-hero frown, but he's fighting back a grin.

He'd sent the poster, I'm told, to Kathi at college—for

her dorm room wall. It was to be a warning, half-serious, to predatory boys. **Back off, bozos, unless you want to deal with this!** Kathi had looked at the poster, blushed, and stuck it in her closet.

Now it hangs on the hospital room wall opposite the dying Heinz. That photo does not mock his present body, maimed and wasted. Oh, no. It is mirroring his spirit, still larger than life.

Lying there facing it, Heinz is joking with me about the unknown.

"Nobody will tell me what's going to happen!" he gripes. "Not doctors, not anybody."

"Well," I say, "here's my guess. Your kidneys have quit, so toxins are going to build up. And you'll slip into the deepest, most restful sleep you've ever had."

"That's not bad," says Heinz. "What then?"

"I can't promise you anything, buddy," I say. "But my guess—my hope—is that you're in for some fine surprises. I think the first surprise you'll get will be understanding. You'll say, 'Well, I'll be damned! So *that's* what life was all about.'

"And when you know," I add, "phone back, will you?" Heinz begins to laugh—a deep, throaty, wicked chuckle.

"You'd crap yourself!" he growls. Then Heinz laughs some more.

We All Live in a Hundred-Acre Wood

Four years ago, our Friends of the Library program for kids was arranged by Fly Creek's Sarah Wilcox (Nat and Stephanie's mom), who also did some fine reading at it herself. If your Friends group does a similar program next year, you should rouse your inner child and go along. Listen and watch. Hearing the stories is great; watching the little kids, even better.

When my turn came, I read from a book that delighted me the first time I heard it. (I remember the footstool where I sat, chin on hands on knees.) More delight came when I could read it to myself, seated on the floor in the angle between bookcase and fireplace, the world walled out by my father's overstuffed chair.

It was *Winnie the Pooh*. I fell in love early with all its characters. And, without knowing the word for it, I fell in love with its tone. (Tone, as I learned a long time later, is the part of language that projects the speaker's attitude— toward his subject, his audience, and himself.)

The tone of the Pooh stories is entrancing. For we're really just listening in. The stories are told, not to us, but to a very young Christopher Robin; told by a father who both loves and delights in his little boy. He builds his whimsical stories around the boy's stuffed animals, and works Christopher Robin into the plots, as well.

As the stories unfold, many of them include bits of dialog between boy and dad. The child's questions and his dad's answers glow with a trust and loving warmth that can still touch grown-up boys and girls, even after they've gone gray-haired and perhaps a little deaf.

One modern reprint of *Winnie the Pooh* shows a fine photo of the original stuffed Pooh in Christopher Robin's lap, and him in his father's. But the photo shows the whimsy of the senior Milne. He has shrunk back as if hiding behind boy and bear, and shaped his thin features to stare as if he's been discovered and is ready to bolt. The wit in the photo, the implied conspiracy among bear, boy, and man, are woven right into the book's tone.

But besides the tone of *Winnie the Pooh*, of course I loved the characters. A. A. Milne has written classic fables, putting our human traits into his animals. Through them, we can understand humans all the better. Kids especially love these animals, I think, because they mostly embody our human weaknesses.

There is Owl with his baseless pretensions of deep knowledge. (He can, says an ironic Milne, even spell his own name, W-O-L.) Owl has all the other animals fooled about his wisdom, and perhaps even himself.

There is Piglet, who thinks of himself as A Very Small Animal and usually feels vulnerable, put-upon, overlooked. Piglet, always scared of vague dangers, but scared to look scared, too.

There's dear Pooh, the Bear of Very Little Brain. Laboring to think clearly, to hold on to a subject, but so easily distracted by the more mundane, especially the thought of food. Pooh, given to grand pronouncements, hoping mightily no one will ask him to explain. Pooh, so often blundering into trouble, but so creative in explaining away his defeats, to others and to himself.

And there's my very favorite. (Is he yours?) It's Eeyore the donkey: gloomy, depressed, and relishing every minute of it. Eeyore of the hanging head, who demands steady sympathy from the other animals. When he's slighted, he feels even more gloomy—and even more pleased that his grim view has been confirmed.

And then there are Kanga and Roo, and Rabbit and all his friends and relations. And the never-seen but always threatening woozles and heffalump. All these creatures populated my childhood, and somehow made humans and the world easier to grasp.

And myself easier to grasp, as well. For shadowy fears sometimes faded when I thought of Pooh and Piglet on the hunt, circling a big bush and shaken by the increasing number of footprints they were following. Or of Piglet alone, trying to screw up his courage to look into the heffalump trap.

And, besides realizing that I shared the world with people very much like Pooh and his friends, over a lifetime I've come to see something more. I'm all those animals, too.

I've a Pooh in me, blundering about, trying to think large thoughts, making pronouncements I hope won't be challenged. And I'm sometimes a Piglet, quailing in front of imaginary dangers, or figuratively jumping up and down to squeak, "I'm here! What about me?"

Certainly I catch myself being WOL, trying to sound more clever than I'll ever be. And I've more than a streak of Eeyore in me, too; ready to see the worst in things, to be happy being sad.

Sometimes when I face myself in the morning mirror, I quote Eeyore when the other animals, who've trekked to his Gloomy Place to cheer him up, greet him with bright hullos. I address my bleary-eyed self with Eeyore's response. I use the donkey's words but, I hope, A. A. Milne's tone, so gentle, so accepting of imperfect life.

"Oh," I mutter. "Hullo. Lost your way?"

Back Among the Unaware

I'm cheating in this column, writing it far ahead of the time when it will be apt. At least I think that's so; I can't know. But I do know that, though I'm still sailing along (albeit low in the water), fog banks lie ahead. Inevitably, my time will come to slip back among the Earth's creatures that, though living, are doing so without abstract "introspection"; without the capacity to "look inside" and say, to themselves, much less others, "Hey, here I am! I'm alive and aware of it. I'm living and I KNOW IT!"

Carrots can't do that, nor canaries, nor dahlias, lions, crabgrass, oysters, oak trees, dung beetles, eagles, mushrooms, eagles, or plankton. Nor, for that matter, can the dear old planet itself, cart wheeling through space but unaware, dreamlessly asleep. It shrugs sometimes in its sleep; it rumbles, vents, crumples, or floods its skin in ways that terrify us who crawl over it. But neither the rolling ball of rock itself nor any mountain, stone or grain of sand of it, is alive, much less aware of itself.

We humans are. For beyond physical bodies, senses, emotions, even imagination (which we share, to varying degrees with all the living), we can also think. We can take inchoate sense impressions, add them to constantly changing imagination, and then do something no other species can (at least in a way we understand): we can form ideas, string them into sequences. We can think. We have, in short, a mind.

Back in the college classroom, I used to startle students by saying that they'd been constantly talking to themselves, by day and probably by night, since the dawn of their consciousness. "And," I'd add, "if you've just said to yourself, 'That's crap! I don't talk to myself,' you've just proved my point," They'd frown, then pause, grin, laugh.

Next I'd remind them that, not only could they think, but they could think about their ability to think—as they were then doing right then. (Furrowed brows.) And further, that they could think about their capacity to think about thinking—as they were then doing. (Pained expressions.) I knew I could push it further, but their heads would start to hurt.

Thought is (I think) that endless internal monologue, wondrously revved up by our ability to give names to things and actions, states of being, plus their qualities and relations. Because we've a brain evolved enough to make and juggle words, we can speak to ourselves and to others with amazing sophistication. We've even developed ways to record our thoughts and so giving them a seeming permanence.

Now, among his myriad of thoughts, any maturing human finally arrives at an especially sobering one: This miraculous ability to scan the world, then speak about it to oneself and even to others, will eventually decay and die, perhaps ahead of our physical beings. We even have a word for it: dementia, "unthinkingness."

In that future I won't be writing any letters, or saying anything, or having any clear perception of myself, the world, my God. My Parkinson's Plus (whatever kind it turns out to be) will have taken away intellect, and with it all powers of awareness, recognizing, naming, defining, analyzing, evaluating. I'll be like my brother animals in other species, perhaps an almost-insensate animal like an oyster, or like a vegetable. We know that grim term, "vegetative state." Eventually, that's to be my state; and it's about that time that I'm writing to you now, against a time when I can't.

What will that limbo be like? Well, there's no knowing

now, any more than there will be then. For all knowing will have been put gently aside, replaced, perhaps, by a kind of sleep. One hopes it's untroubled by dreams.

Some wit said, "Thought of one's approaching execution marvelously focuses the mind." And the thought of becoming un-minded can shake us to our souls. To be set back among the other animals or, worse, into a vegetative state? What kind of life would that be? What purpose would it have? Of what use would it be to be me?

That last question is, I think, the telling one. If I'm no longer of use to myself (because I'm unconscious of me), then what possible meaning will my continued life have?

A useful answer is at the end of T. S. Eliot's *Murder in the Cathedral.* At that point in the drama, the powerful have done their sacrilege inside the great cathedral; and the next morning (and for all mornings after) the humble folk of Canterbury are about their usual lives. Scrubbers and sweepers are in the cathedral square, and, as they work, Eliot has them sing an astounding hymn of praise.

They remind themselves that ALL earthly creations praise God, Who brought them to being, simply by their being. "They affirm Thee in living; all things affirm Thee in living; the bird in the air, both the hawk and the finch; the beast on the earth, both the wolf and the lamb ..."

Then comes a statement of the human role: "Therefore man, whom Thou hast made to be conscious of Thee, must consciously praise Thee, in thought and word and deed." And, mind you, not only in our own name! For we are part of the planet and all that lives on it, no less for our vaunted consciousness. One with creation, we are meant to be its voice, lifted in praise for all of it, ourselves included.

And what of when we can no longer consciously praise, when our voices have stopped, cognition failed? Well, we slip back among the unaware, who praise simply by their continued living, their continuing to exist, *to be.*

But we humans have, even then, a further function, a cosmic usefulness right inside the human family.

Once I told a Quaker friend that I regretted the time when I'd be beyond any kind of giving. His answer: "Jim, that's when yours becomes a ministry of receiving." He said that there can't be loving givers without receivers, whether the latter are conscious or unaware. Both givers and receivers are needed in the great economy of growth toward God.

And so, a new role lies ahead for me—and, of course, eventually for you. It's a humbling one but still a part of that great, divine economy. Humbly accepted, it can raise us above our deadening egoism. And, even if we're reduced to an oyster's awareness or beyond, we're still useful receivers of others' loving service, still helping raise them toward God.

I like that thought. To that I say, Amen!

Epilogue:

"Tidings of Comfort and Joy"

*This epilogue was written as a column a dozen Decembers
ago, but it seems to belong right here to thank you for
wobbling along beside me to this book's end.*

Maybe I've already had my best Christmas gift. If so, I don't
mind. It was a great one.

This year the Cooperstown, New York Rotary Club
decided to go caroling. The plan was to board a bus at the
Otesaga hotel, sing at several nursing homes, and then
return to the Otesaga for a Christmas buffet. My Rotarian
wife signed up, and I got to go along as a spouse.

Rotary clubs are usually a pretty good cross-section of
an area's movers and shakers. That's certainly true here, and
the Cooperstown club approached the project with zest.
Gerry Phelan headed a committee that split up the tasks.
Joan Badgley booked the bus and laid out the route. With
Rotary funds, Susan Streek bought and then wrapped two
hundred token gifts. Bob Schlather (who besides lawyer's
skills, has a fine baritone) planned the music. Jim Woolson,
a one-man press gang, signed up the singers.

When we boarded the bus at five-thirty, a cold drizzle
had turned into heavy, steady snow; but we waded through
it into each of our gigs. Bob Schlather led us on like King
Wenceslaus himself, followed by two dozen pages.

At the sites we were greeted warmly by staff, who'd
gathered audiences for us in brightly decorated day rooms.

In each we'd sing a handful of carols, then exit to "We Wish You a Merry Christmas!" and a patter of soft applause.

We'd climb back into the bus, brushing off snow, chattering, laughing. Then we'd roll along through the snow-covered streets, singing more carols just for fun.

Mostly, the singers were women and men in the early middle years of their lives and professions. They were full of good health, energy, and success. And, as they rode along, they were warmed by a sense of doing something good and apt.

At each stop though, the carolers carried their intense vitality into a setting that quietly contradicted it—in among lives whose drive had ebbed, drained away by age or failed health.

That sharp contrast struck others and me, I think, most strongly at The Meadows, our county's nursing facility. There we sang our way through the decorated corridors, then formed up and sang out fully wherever residents had been gathered into public rooms.

Many among whom we stood singing were aware and grateful, even joined in. Others gazed into the distance, perhaps raising images of Christmases long past. And some, lost in private twilight, knit their brows as if displeased. This sudden noisiness and movement distracted them from getting hold of it. Of that illusive whatever-it-is. That important thing that must be considered or done, but that always drifted just beyond grasp.

The singers, I think, all caught the bittersweet contrast, standing there with melting snow on their shoulders, cheeks still rosy from the outside cold. As they sang they read their futures—a good thing, as Scrooge found out, to do at Christmas.

Good for them I say! Good for those Rotarians who had borrowed time from their busy lives—and who faced up, that night, to more than the cold.

And good for that one ancient, sunken-cheeked man,

somewhere deep in The Meadows, who gave me my best Christmas gift.

In bathrobe and pajamas, he sat strapped loosely in a wheelchair, slumped against its tipped back, head rolled to the side. His eyes were closed, face slack. Asleep, I thought, or past all knowing.

But when we ended "God Rest Ye, Merry Gentlemen," there was slight movement in that face. As we sang the last three words, the man's lips formed them. "Comfort and Joy."

Thank you, sir. And Merry Christmas.

And God rest you, my friend, for walking along with me.
May He save you from dismay.
May yours be comfort and joy.
Always.

About the Author

A Maryland native, **Jim Atwell** spent thirteen years as a Catholic teaching monk in the Christian Brothers religious order. In 1969, he returned to life as a layman and took a faculty position at Anne Arundel Community College near his hometown of Annapolis. In his twenty-three years at the College, he served as assistant, associate, and full professor, and as chairman, dean, and Vice-President for Academic Affairs. In retirement, he is an emeritus member of the Anne Arundel faculty. His personal spiritual development now marks him as being a practicing Quaker for forty years.

Jim owes his deep love of Upstate New York to his late first wife Gwen, who grew up near Cooperstown. After her death in 1989, he moved north to start life again in the 18th-century farmhouse they had bought for a retirement home. In 1997 Jim remarried; he and Anne Geddes-Atwell still make their home in Fly Creek, raising sheep and chickens, and pursuing writing and graphic design, respectively.

Jim's award-winning weekly columns in Cooperstown's two weekly papers have been a regional institution for a dozen years. They are followed by thousands of readers in print, and thousands more on *The Cooperstown Crier* website. The New York State Press Association has recognized his writing eight times with awards for content and style. Newspaper writing led to a recent anthology of his columns, *From Fly Creek: Celebrating Life in Leatherstocking Country*, published by North Country Books in 2005.

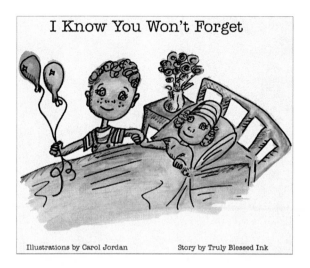

I Know You Won't Forget

Illustrations by Carol Jordan   Story by Truly Blessed Ink

I Know You Won't Forget is the story of a young boy whose mother suffers a traumatic brain injury. After being embarrassed by her unreliable behavior and ridiculed by his classmates, the boy helps his mother develop some coping strategies to overcome her impairments, ultimately finding happiness. The story shows children how a brain injury can affect everyone in a family and strain relationships, and how resulting issues can be resolved. **Written and illustrated by a group of brain injury survivors in Upstate New York.**

I Know You Won't Forget
Story by Truly Blessed Ink; Illustrations by Carol Jordan
$16.95 retail; ISBN: 978-0-9789066-1-0
40 pages, 10" x 8", full color, casewrap hardcover
Suitable for ages 8 and up

CPSIA information can be obtained at www.ICGtesting.com
Printed in the USA
LVOW071658111211

258911LV00001B/87/P